D0405539

WHY DIETS FAIL

WHY
DIETS
FAIL

(Because You're Addicted to Sugar)

Science Explains How to
End Cravings, Lose Weight,
and Get Healthy

Nicole M. Avena, PhD, and John R. Talbott

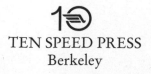

TEN SPEED PRESS
Berkeley

Disclaimer: The information contained in this book is based on the experience and research of the authors. It is not intended as a substitute for consulting with your physician or other health-care provider. Any attempt to diagnose and treat an illness should be done under the direction of a health-care professional. The publisher and authors are not responsible for any adverse effects or consequences resulting from the use of any of the suggestions, preparations, or procedures discussed in this book.

Copyright © 2014 by Dr. Nicole M. Avena and John R. Talbott

All rights reserved.

Published in the United States by Ten Speed Press, an imprint of the Crown Publishing Group, a division of Random House LLC, a Penguin Random House Company, New York.
www.crownpublishing.com
www.tenspeed.com

Ten Speed Press and the Ten Speed Press colophon are registered trademarks of Random House LLC

Library of Congress Cataloging-in-Publication Data
Avena, Nicole M., 1978–
    Why diets fail (because you're addicted to sugar) : science explains how to end cravings, lose weight, and get healthy / Nicole M. Avena, PhD. and John R. Talbott. — First edition.
        pages cm
1. Sugar-free diet. 2. Sugar—Physiological effect. 3. Reducing diets. 4. Health.
I. Talbott, John R., 1955– II. Title. III. Title: Why diets fail (because you are addicted to sugar).
    RM237.85.A94 2013
    613.2'8332—dc23

                                                                                    2013021488

Hardcover ISBN: 978-1-60774-486-3
eBook ISBN: 978-1-60774-487-0

Printed in the United States of America

Design by Katy Brown
Cover photography by Katie Newburn

Illustrations on page 47: (from left) ©istock.com/gresei, ©istock.com/ansonsaw, ©istock.com/pinstock, ©istock.com/SKrow, and ©istock.com/evemilla; page 160: (dog) ©istock.com/alashi, (dog bowl) ©istock.com/HitToon, and (bell) ©istock .com/lushik; and on page 161: (food) ©istock.com/appleuzr and (faces) ©istock.com/ PinkTag.

10 9 8 7 6 5 4 3 2 1

First Edition

To SAB

—NICOLE M. AVENA

To Gary Taubes

—JOHN R. TALBOTT

Contents

Acknowledgments // viii

Introduction // 1

PART ONE

HOW SUGAR CAUSES YOU TO OVEREAT

STEP 1
Why Your Past Diet Attempts Have Failed // 17

STEP 2
Weigh In on Your Sugar Intake // 32

STEP 3
The New Science of Sugar Addiction // 58

PART TWO

HOW TO OVERCOME YOUR ADDICTION TO SUGAR

STEP 4

The Sugar Freedom Plan for Breaking
Your Addiction // 84

STEP 5

What to Eat and What *Not* to Eat // 118

STEP 6

Managing Your Withdrawal // 140

STEP 7

Managing Your Cravings // 152

STEP 8

Avoiding a Relapse
(and What to Do If One Occurs) // 165

CONCLUSION

How to Maintain Your New,
Addiction-Free Way of Eating // 175

Appendix: Sugar Equivalency Table // 195

Resources // 208

Endnotes // 212

Index // 225

Acknowledgments

There are many important people to thank and acknowledge in the development of this book. We especially thank our editor, Julie Bennett, and the entire team at Ten Speed Press, as well as the folks at the Crown Publishing Group and Random House, for their assistance and support in the writing and development of this book.
—Nicole M. Avena and John R. Talbott

I would like to thank all of my colleagues and collaborators for their research as well as the valuable information that they have produced in the fields of nutrition, neuroscience, and addiction. There are too many of you to name, but I value each of your unique contributions to our field. I would like to thank Bart Hoebel for his mentorship and friendship, and for getting me involved and excited about appetite research. I would also like to thank Susan Murray for her invaluable efforts assisting with the research, organization, and development of this book. She was there at every step along the way, and her interest in and enthusiasm for this project significantly contributed to the final product. I would also like to thank Cindy Kroll and Monica Gordillo for their assistance with researching various aspects of the contents in this book. In addition, I thank my friends and family for their help and support along the way. I am blessed to have an amazing network of loving and supportive friends. I especially thank Nicole, Nicki, Beth, and Marylynn for their encouragement while working on this project. I extend my gratitude to my parents and siblings (both the A team and the B team) for cheering me on. I also owe an infinite amount of thanks to my husband, Eamon. You've supported me unrelentingly during this project, as well as all of the other little projects that I have concocted in life and work, which inevitably develop into something much, much bigger than anticipated. Your advice, levelheadedness, and comic relief provide the glue that keeps me together. Bert, thanks for staying up late with me all of those nights. Also, last but not least, thank you Stella for your patience and understanding and for allowing my work to temporarily encroach on our playtime. I love you all dearly.

—Nicole

I would like to thank my friends and family who had to put up with my withdrawal symptoms when I went on this diet. Thanks especially to Teresa, who was an early guinea pig and who demonstrated that the diet really did make one feel dramatically better, more at ease, and more connected with life. I would like to thank Becky for her great job transcribing and proofing the book, Dottie for delivering on her promises as always, and Bill, Mario, Roberto, Tacho, Jacinto, Luis, and all the other usual suspects at K-38 for making the writing of this book as enjoyable as catching the perfect wave.

—John

Introduction

*"Americans have more food to eat than any other
people and more diets to keep them from eating it."*

—YOGI BERRA

L ook around you. The vast majority of people in the United
States are overweight, and a growing number are obese. Rich,
poor, old, young, male, female—we see obesity happening across
all social domains, races, and ages. Body-weight problems aren't
restricted to certain groups of people. Right now, more than 60 percent of Americans are overweight, and more than 30 percent are
obese.[1] And these numbers are projected to continue to rise. In fact,
by 2030, researchers have predicted that 42 percent of Americans
will be obese.[2] This is not just something that is occurring within
the United States either; the obesity epidemic is a global problem.

Although many of us may want to lose weight simply to
improve our appearance or how we feel about ourselves, there are
important medical reasons for controlling body weight. Excess body
weight has been associated with a number of health risks, including
cancer, heart disease, and diabetes. Despite these potential harmful

consequences and public health warnings regarding the dangers of obesity, many people continue to overeat. And this isn't hard to do. High-calorie, high-sugar food is easily accessible to many people today, and portion sizes have increased dramatically over the years. Food is also a big part of our social lives and, as you will read in later chapters, has taken on a new role in our society.

It didn't used to be this way. Fifty years ago, it was much less common to see fat people and usually a rarity to see fat children. So, what happened to cause such an abrupt and dramatic change in the waistline of society? Certainly, social factors made it easier to stay slim fifty years ago. There were more stay-at-home moms to prepare healthy, wholesome, homemade meals; more people smoked cigarettes (which are appetite suppressants); and, importantly, there weren't as many food choices or the large portions we have today.

Despite these societal changes, lots of things have happened in the past fifty years that would lead one to think that we should be *healthier*, not heavier. There have been dramatic advances in the diagnosis and treatment of diseases, like cancer and heart disease. We have learned an incredible amount from scientists about ways in which we can live healthier, longer lives. And we have so many luxuries that should make losing weight and staying well easy: We have twenty-four-hour gyms, a variety of health food stores and healthy food choices, and even an array of "diet" foods and programs that are supposed to help us keep our body weight in check. Low-fat, low-carb, no-carb—there are so many different plans out there that you could spend a lifetime trying them all. Dieting is a multibillion-dollar industry. With all of the books, magazine articles, and television programs focused on weight loss, it is really a wonder how overeating could be such a looming problem, not only in the United States but throughout the world.

Why is this happening? Why can't people just stop eating so much and lose weight? Many possible culprits have been identified.

Sure, people are stressed and lead relatively sedentary lifestyles, and this undoubtedly contributes to the problem of overeating. Also, genetics play a role; overweight people will give their genes (and thus perhaps a tendency to be overweight) to their children, and they might also raise them in a home that promotes excess food intake or unhealthy eating habits. But there is more to it than just these factors.

Science has told us that the answer is simple: exercise, minimize stress, and eat right. It's the *eating right* part of the solution where things get complicated. In response to the public interest in being healthy and losing weight, a plethora of diet books and programs were developed. Many of these offer sound, practical advice that, on paper, looks great. Many of the diet programs out there *should* work, but they don't. People go on a diet and then quit; weight regain and yo-yo dieting have become a common, vicious cycle for too many Americans. The problem is adherence. People just can't stick to the prescribed plan, whatever it may be.

Perhaps there is another factor that could hold the key to reducing overeating for many people—something that would help to explain why people often feel drawn to certain types of foods, crave them, and can't seem to eat them in moderation. (Recall that famous Lay's potato chip commercial: "Bet you can't eat just one.") Could food be *addictive*? Is there something about the foods that we tend to overeat that makes us addicted to them and leads us to continue to overindulge?

The crux of this book is this: Diets fail for a very simple reason. The key to losing weight may be to eliminate excess calories, which we undoubtedly get in the form of added sugars and excessive amounts of other carbohydrates in our diet. But if you are psychologically and chemically dependent on these types of foods, your "addiction" may lead you into a vicious cycle of overeating, withdrawal, and craving for these foods, which can derail your attempts to cut back on intake and lose weight, and ultimately lead to continued overeating and weight gain.

How Did This Book Come to Be?

Before we get into the details of how and why foods, and sugars in particular, can be addictive—and how you can overcome this addiction—we would like to tell you the story of how this book came to be. It is quite an interesting story, as we are two people on different coasts, in different careers, on very different life paths, who have come together through a series of events that were prompted by our mutual interest in trying to understand why controlling the intake of certain foods can be so difficult for some individuals.

JOHN'S STORY

I never thought I would write a diet book. But last year, I realized my weight had ballooned up to 252 pounds, which by medical standards meant that, at 6'2", I was not only overweight but borderline obese.

I always thought I carried my weight rather well. I rationalized by telling myself that I was just big-boned and had good, strong legs. I knew I wasn't thin, but I didn't realize how fat I had become. When I looked at pictures, I didn't recognize myself. Photos for my driver's license and passport didn't look like me but rather some inflated version of me, like I was a giant balloon character floating along in the Macy's Thanksgiving Day Parade.

Then I discovered Gary Taubes and a piece he wrote for the *New York Times Magazine* entitled "Is Sugar Toxic?"[3] That led me to his excellent book *Why We Get Fat: And What to Do About It.*[4]

I learned that consuming excess amounts of sugars and starches is fattening and toxic. The more I read and thought about it, the more I began to wonder whether sugar could be addictive. Addiction is something I am familiar with. I have spent much of my adult life researching and trying to figure out the causes of addiction, because I have had a problem with alcohol over the years. If sugar and starches are also addictive and cause people to get fat, this is something that I'm interested in.

So, I decided to stop eating sugar and most fast-digesting starches. And I can tell you, it was not easy, but the results I saw are just short of amazing. The fact that most diet books make similar claims of incredible outcomes cheapens what I am about to tell you, because what I experienced after cutting out sugar was truly life changing. Six months after adopting this sugar-free way of eating, I had lost 52 pounds. I went from 252 pounds to 200 pounds. But that's not the full story. Three months into my experiment, I no longer felt lousy every day. I really started feeling good for the first time that I could remember. I mean really good. I mean jumping out of bed in the morning before the alarm clock rang with no need for caffeine or other stimulants. I mean wanting to exercise and play sports not because I was supposed to but rather because I actually enjoyed it. Mostly, I must admit vainly, I took great pleasure in knowing that my body more resembled the tight-muscled look it had when I was a national champion rower at Cornell in 1977 than the bulbous, fatty blob it had become by the time I was fifty-seven.

Because I wasn't eating carbs or sugar, I necessarily had to eat more protein, and eating protein and engaging in regular exercise are both great for adding muscle and definition to your body. I had lost enormous amounts of fat throughout my body—especially in my stomach, chest, and buttocks area—but I was also simultaneously adding muscle weight. And since muscle weighs more than the same volume of fat, my weight loss felt even more meaningful: the numbers on the scale kept going down despite adding dense muscle to my body. I went from a 39-inch pant size to a 35-inch pant size. Four inches may not sound like a huge reduction to you, but consider that now, with a 35-inch waist, I am only five inches away from the smallest pant size Costco even carries anymore. And this is from someone who is 6'2" tall.

This diet did something else rather amazing for me. It made me feel so good about myself that it changed the way I interacted with people. Before, I was constantly going through many mini withdrawals throughout the day whenever I didn't have my sugar fix, and with these mini withdrawals came a level of anxiety that led me to be short-tempered, with little patience for others. Bottom line, I wasn't always fun to be around. Now, I find myself smiling as I walk down the street. I find pleasure in simple things. I love to catch a beautiful wave to surf or to see a seal or dolphin pop up next to me in the water just to say hello. I enjoy making a simple pass in soccer that allows an open teammate to score a goal. I know it sounds mushy and trite, but that is the degree of change that I've felt in my personal life with this diet plan. Yes, losing weight is part of it, along with the return of self-esteem that comes from being more fit, but the big difference is eliminating a substance from my system that can be so addictive that I may constantly be suffering these mini withdrawals between doses.

I can certainly attest to sugar's addictiveness. When I quit eating sugar and starches, I went through a nasty withdrawal period that lasted two to three weeks with symptoms that were very similar to the flu. I had headaches, anxiety, nausea, muscle aches and pains, and even nightmares. After that, I had a lingering feeling of discomfort that lasted two to three months. I wasn't in pain, so to speak; these symptoms resided more in my mind than in my body. But it wasn't necessarily fun either. One of the traits that addictive substances and addictive behaviors have in common is that they can both stimulate the brain to overproduce certain neurochemicals, which can lead to feelings of euphoria. Once you stop consuming an addictive substance like sugar (or nicotine or alcohol), not only does the brain quit overproducing these chemicals, but it is also not uncommon for the brain to then underproduce them, thus leading to the opposite of euphoria: depression. But, actually, all of this pain and melancholy was a good sign. It meant that my body was cleansing itself, and I eventually realized that the negative effects would be temporary. Like most people, I can put up with slight amounts of discomfort as long as I know I will not be subjected to them permanently and that there is a purpose to the pain that makes it worth enduring.

It took me approximately six months to realize what I had accomplished. It wasn't just the weight loss. What became most incredible over time was that, unlike other diets, this change in my life is permanent and I feel little risk that I will relapse and resume my old habits. It is this sense of permanence, especially in light of all my prior failed attempts to lose weight, that most impressed me and made me realize that this very low-sugar and low-starch diet was truly extraordinary and unique. I felt as if I were sitting on a magic cure. In the United States, millions of adults are overweight or obese. What was I to do with my newfound knowledge?

Well, even though I am not a nutritionist or an addiction expert, it turns out I am an author, so I wanted to write a book to tell others about what I had discovered. I have spent twenty years of my adult life contemplating and writing about some very big ideas in the areas of finance, global economics, and even the promotion of democracy and freedom. I have been lucky enough to write books and research articles that have been helpful in understanding how our global economy operates and the dangers we face when we allow too much power to reside in the hands of a few. But I believe that nothing I have worked on to this point is as important as the concepts presented in this book. Sure, we would all like to lose weight and be fitter, but the importance of the approach in this book is in how it will help you reawaken your passion for life and feel reconnected with friends and family once the adverse consequences of consuming sugar are eliminated. Though I wanted to write this book, I knew, however, that I would need help from someone who has expertise in the areas of food intake, nutrition, and addiction. Determined, I decided to contact the top addiction experts in the country to see if my ideas and experience were backed by current science and research. That is how I came to learn of Dr. Avena's work in nutrition and addiction.

Dr. Avena has made a career of studying why people like to eat, or not eat, food. She studies the psychological foundations and brain mechanisms that lead people to make decisions about how much,

Dr. Avena's Research

As a scientist and research psychologist, I study and try to understand the microscopic details of the neurotransmitters and brain receptors involved in the process of eating. Understanding the minute chemical changes in the brain that explain why people like certain foods, and sometimes choose to eat them in excess, has clear implications for obesity and some eating disorders, as well as for many of the people out there who are just trying to lose weight.

In recent years, the obesity epidemic has become one of the most important problems faced by our society. Because of this, many researchers are working diligently to figure out why and how so many people are becoming overweight or obese. I have taken a new approach to studying obesity by blending the disciplines of neuroscience, psychology, nutrition, and addiction. Studies from my laboratory and others suggest that overeating and obesity can produce behaviors and changes in the brain that look like a drug addiction. But we aren't addicted to drugs; we are addicted to high-calorie, high-sugar foods.

and what type of, food to eat. She had been doing important studies to answer a burning question: Could it be that so many people are overweight or obese because they are "addicted" to foods like sugars? So, I wrote a short email to her asking if she thought my diet ideas were novel and valid. To my delight, she responded with one of the most incredible emails I have received in my lifetime.

First, she said there was nothing in my conjectures about sugar's addictiveness that was counter to any research she knew of. Second, she told me about all of the different ways that she has been testing the hypothesis that sugar could be addictive in the lab. Her research group has conducted a series of experiments with lab rats, and the results suggested that when rats voluntarily ate excessive amounts of sugars, they began, in many ways, to resemble addicts. The idea that certain foods might be addictive was, and still is, a new area of scientific exploration, and one that might hold the answers to a lot of unanswered questions.

Here was someone I had never met who had come to some of the same conclusions that I had, not through personal experience like myself, but through rigorous scientific research in the lab. It was incredibly validating and reassuring to hear that my experience was not an anomaly, and that there is a whole line of scientific research focused on understanding why and how overeating sugars could cause weight gain and promote addiction.

The end result was that Dr. Avena and I decided to combine our unique experiences with the addictive nature of sugars and coauthor this book. I jumped at the chance to work with her, and what a great experience this collaboration has been for me. But there is a huge benefit to you, the reader, from our collaboration as well.

Why You Need to Read *This* "Diet" Book

These days, diet books are a dime a dozen, but few books combine the lived experience of someone who has implemented that diet and seen amazing results with the scientific research that supports and explains why the eating plan works. In *Why Diets Fail*, you gain all the latest scientific knowledge and expertise from Dr. Avena, who has a PhD in psychology and neuroscience and is an expert in the fields of addiction, nutrition, and obesity, informed by insights from John, who has lived through this experience.

Moreover, you will learn about some fascinating research discoveries that you may not yet be aware of, many of which may explain why certain approaches that you have taken in the past to lose weight have been unsuccessful. All too often, research findings are reported in scholarly journals or discussed among researchers and members of the scientific community, and even though they may have direct application to human life, they rarely reach the larger public. Thus, such findings fail to have a significant effect on the day-to-day lives of the people who could benefit. That's why this book is so valuable. Together, we'll explain why John's revelation, and resolution, regarding addiction to sugars was beneficial to his life, and could be to yours, in so many ways.

Although diet will certainly be discussed, we're reticent to call this a "diet" book, as that term doesn't necessarily reflect how extremely valuable this book can be to individuals who struggle to achieve and maintain a healthy body weight. But trust us, when you implement the diet, like John did, you can reawaken to a life that is more fulfilling, fun, and rewarding than anything you could have imagined.

Treating Food as a Drug

One important shortcoming of most diets out there is that they fail to recognize that highly palatable, highly caloric foods can be addictive. And when we say "addictive," we don't mean in the fun-loving sense like "I am addicted to watching *CSI*" or "I am addicted to checking my Facebook." In this context, we use the term "addicted" more literally.

The idea that food, and sugars in particular, have addictive characteristics is not necessarily new. For many years, we've heard reports of people claiming they feel driven to eat sugars and other sweets, much as drug addicts might feel compelled to get their next fix. These stories, while fascinating, were largely anecdotal. Yet studies now suggest that foods high in added sugars and other carbohydrates satisfy the clinical and scientific requirements for an addictive substance, like a drug that's abused. Excessive intake of some types of foods can result in behaviors and changes in the brain that are akin to what one would see with addiction to drugs. Yes—heroin, morphine, cocaine, alcohol . . . and sugars.

Studies suggest that people who are clinically addicted to food can be found among people who are overweight, obese, or normal weight, so addiction to food is not necessarily something that is exclusive to obesity. People with disrupted eating patterns, such as binge eating disorder, may also meet the criteria for addiction to food. However, another important group that may be affected by the addictive nature of food is made up of those *at risk* for becoming addicted—and that group includes almost all of us.

As we'll discuss later on, addiction is a multifaceted disorder that has multiple causes. Genetics certainly play a role, but so does the environment. Repeated exposure to, and use of, one's particular drug of abuse promotes addiction. Think about what it would be like if it were easier to obtain drugs like cocaine or heroin—if they were legal and socially accepted, and we were bombarded constantly with pictures of people enjoying them—the drug problem in this country would undoubtedly be worse than it already is. Because our modern-day food environment *is* dominated by high-sugar and high-carbohydrate foods, we are *all* at risk for developing an addiction. So, even if you don't feel compelled to overeat sugar-rich foods, and you don't experience other symptoms of dependence, you can still benefit from this book. While this science is relatively new, it has far-reaching implications not only for you as an individual who may be struggling to lose weight but also for multiple disciplines, including public health and policy regarding the marketing and sale of certain types of foods. (We'll say more about this in later chapters.)

How do we get addicted? There are several ways. One relates back to the idea we mentioned at the start of the chapter about how we have more food choices now than we did fifty years ago. While in many ways the assortment of foods available to us is an advantage (as the saying goes, variety is the spice of life), the variety of foodstuffs out there are not all healthy. We are plagued with fast-food restaurants, convenience food stores, and snack machines pretty much wherever we go. Even in the grocery store, we are faced with aisles of different types of snack foods and treats, cakes, cookies, and sweets. And we buy these items up. Not only do we like to eat them, but often, to "save money," we also buy them in massive quantities at shopping clubs or in value packs. Those supersized bags of chips, sodas, and other snacks may be adding to our supersized waistlines. And this type of excess eating doesn't just apply to junk food. Other foods, some of which are promoted as being healthy, are being consumed in excess. For example, bagels, boxes of cereal, and loaves of bread have, like us, become larger and larger over time.

Why do we keep buying and eating such foods? Well, for one, they are easy to obtain, as so often they are right there in front of us.

Our fast-paced modern-day lifestyles, which have left us with less time to prepare meals at home, have forced us to become dependent on this convenience.

However, dependence on food appears to be more than just a matter of convenience; science suggests that we are biologically dependent on certain types of foods, and this may contribute to obesity.

What exactly does it mean to be addicted to food? Due to the constant, excessive exposure to foods laden with sugar and other carbohydrates (as well as their logos, commercials, and advertisements) that has occurred as a result of our modern food environment, many of us may experience significant cravings for sugar-containing foods. As we build up tolerance for them over time, it takes larger and larger amounts of those candy bars, chips, and ice cream cones to satisfy our cravings. Most importantly, some of us may experience withdrawal symptoms between sugar fixes, which can be exacerbated when we quit consuming sugars and other carbohydrates for a period of time (if you've ever tried to eat a low-carb diet, you know what we mean). We may also have powerful cravings for these foods when deprived of them, even when this deprivation is self-induced, and these cravings can lead to overeating and excessive calorie intake, which means more weight gain.

Here's an example. Lower-carbohydrate diets have been found to be superior to low-fat diets in terms of promoting weight loss.[5] And most low-carb diets involve reducing or eliminating added sugars and other carbohydrates. But as we mentioned above, when people follow diets like the Atkins Diet and quit eating these high-sugar, high-carb foods, many experience discomforts like headaches, for example.[6] None of us feels good when we have a headache, so who can blame us for cheating a little bit or, in many cases, quitting the diet completely. But these headaches or any of the other discomforts that have been reported by people eating a low-carb diet may actually be signs of withdrawal. These popular diets don't tell you that when you rapidly switch from a diet dominated by carbohydrates to one that lacks them, you may experience the negative feelings and physiological changes that are akin to a drug withdrawal.

Even though it is not a pleasant process to endure, reminiscent of what happens when heroin addicts go into detox, withdrawal from sugars and other carbohydrates is part of the process of no longer being chemically dependent on them. In order to break free of your dependence, you must know how to anticipate and endure the withdrawal and cravings that might lure you back to overeating high-carbohydrate foods. That is the purpose of this book—to offer a new approach toward achieving your weight-loss goals by recognizing and coping with addiction to sugars and other carbohydrates.

How to Use This Book

Why Diets Fail presents an eight-step program to help you lose weight by restricting your intake of certain types of foods, and in some cases eliminating them completely from your diet. At the same time, we understand that adhering to a low-carbohydrate diet needs to be done with an understanding of the possible addictive nature of these types of foods. So we're going to take it slow.

In each chapter, we introduce one new step that is designed to help you learn about your present diet habits, recognize signs of addiction to sugars and other carbohydrates, develop a sensible and realistic low-sugar and low-carbohydrate meal and snack plan, manage your withdrawal and cravings for the carbohydrate-rich foods you lust over, and maintain this way of eating. In the second part of the book, we present the Sugar Freedom Plan, which is a plan for getting you off sugar and on to your new way of eating and living. At the end of each chapter is a section we call Food for

Thought. In these sections, you will be asked to reflect on aspects of your life (your eating patterns, your coping techniques, and other life patterns) so that you can apply the concepts presented in each chapter to *your* life. In addition to these reflections, you may find it helpful to grab a piece of paper and a pencil or pull up a notepad on your handheld device and jot down any information that you find interesting, insightful, and potentially useful for the future as you read the book. You don't have to use complete sentences or reference specific page numbers, you can just write some short phrases or key words that you know will jog your memory. Remember that each one of us is unique and you will be reading this book with your own personal weight-loss and health goals in mind. We provide approximate time frames with regard to reducing or eliminating excess sugar sources from your diet, but these are merely a guide, and you should work through the steps at your own pace.

*

The sad truth is that most of us are overweight because we eat too much. And if you aren't overweight, you are certainly in danger of becoming overweight based on our present food environment. In this book, you will learn about the evidence of food addiction that has been found in both laboratory animals and humans. In addition, you will be given a step-by-step plan that will help you to recognize whether you have an addiction to sugar-rich foods and explain how to reduce your intake of these foods, what foods to eat (or avoid eating), how to cope with the side effects of addiction, and how to reduce behaviors that may lead you back into the cycle of addictive overeating. You will learn ways in which you can replace sugars and other carbohydrates with sensible alternatives that will leave you feeling full and in better control of your weight-loss plan.

Now it's time to get started and take your first step toward a lighter, healthier, sugar-free you.

PART ONE

How Sugar Causes You to Overeat

STEP 1

Why Your Past Diet Attempts Have Failed

"A minute's success pays for the failure of years."

—ROBERT BROWNING, ENGLISH POET

You know from reading the introduction that most diets fail because we're addicted to sugars and carbohydrates. To help you understand overeating from this new angle and to equip you with strategies to break free from the cycle that may be keeping you overweight, it is important to see the common threads that emerge among diet failures. Why do so many of us have difficulty adhering to a healthy diet and maintaining our desired body weight? Understanding why things *don't* work can help you see why the changes you will implement here *will* work, and end up working so well.

The Beginning of the End

As we've discussed, there are a vast number of diets on the market, all of which promise to help us lose weight and keep it off. Yet many of us have cycled on and off diets for the better part of our lives, with one failure after another. These diets clearly don't work; if they did, we wouldn't need to keep trying new ones. Plus, if one of them *really did work*, we would actually lose weight and keep it off, instead of remaining overweight, disappointed, and looking for a better solution.

While we tend to adhere to a particular diet for varying lengths of time, most diets don't last very long. We usually throw in the towel within the first few weeks, often even within the first few days. We start out with determination, hope, and good intentions, so what happens during this time period that leads us right back to where we started? As it turns out, lots of things can happen during this initial dieting period that eventually lead to diet demise.

Normally, things start off well. We are motivated during the first few days. We make a conscious decision to lose weight, and we prepare to start "the diet." Maybe we stock up on or make a mental list of "healthy" foods we plan to eat, or we mark the starting date on the calendar and announce it to our family and friends. Maybe we even enlist a diet partner who also wants to lose weight and get healthy. Those first few days are usually pretty successful, and we may even see a small amount of weight loss, which motivates us to continue.

Unfortunately, things quickly start to unravel. After just a few days, we get sick of eating "diet" foods and bored with the same mundane, flavorless tastes. We find ourselves feeling irritable, cranky, and easily annoyed (which, as you will see later, is probably a manifestation of withdrawal from the sugar-filled and

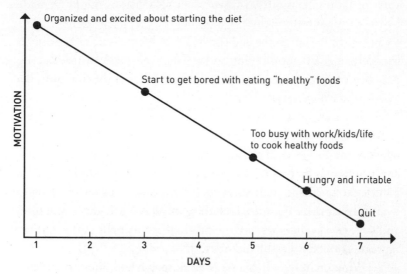

WEEK ONE OF A TYPICAL DIET

Organized and excited about starting the diet

Start to get bored with eating "healthy" foods

Too busy with work/kids/life to cook healthy foods

Hungry and irritable

Quit

MOTIVATION

DAYS

carbohydrate-rich foods that we are accustomed to overeating). The refrigerator stocked with the "diet" foods gets depleted, and other commitments to life, work, and family distract us from our eating plan. Our friend quits the diet (but resolves to start up again next month), so we are left to go it alone. We are hungry and unhappy. The results are slow to appear. It isn't working, so we quit. We say to ourselves, "Maybe this particular diet wasn't the one for me, so I will try a different one." And the vicious cycle starts over again. Does any of this sound familiar?

Who Is to Blame?

Typically, when diets fail, the blame falls on the dieter. People might say that the dieter lacked willpower or that she was lazy. In most cases, the despondent, failed dieter also thinks it is her fault. All sorts of rationalizations, excuses, and explanations might be made by the dieter at first (including blaming the diet itself for her inability to follow it), but in the end the finger of blame is usually pointed squarely at the person trying to lose the weight. And this feeling may be even more pronounced if the failed diet regimen required a lot of physical exercise.

This is not just conjecture; surveys suggest that people believe personal behaviors are the primary reason why so many people are overweight, rather than the amount of junk food available or other environmental factors.[1] However, this commonly held belief is in contrast to scientific evidence, which is finding that societal changes over the past three decades, including our work schedules and food and beverage availability, are the driving factors behind the marked increases in body weight and obesity.

Unfortunately, self-blame is common. Alcoholics are blamed for their lack of resolve, and gamblers are blamed for not having enough self-control and responsibility. But it's not that simple. Science has taught us that personal responsibility is part of a larger, more complicated puzzle, and some things are beyond our personal control. Addiction has a biological basis and is driven, at least in part, by changes in our brains. It can have a powerful influence over our behavior, and it can sabotage our attempts to regulate our behavior.

As a result, failed dieters should not necessarily bear all of the blame. As you will learn in this book, the cause of being overweight is not simply limited to our willpower; other causes may include our biochemistry and the potentially addictive nature of some types of food. Willpower is certainly part of staying on track, and we need to have willpower and dedication to succeed at our health goals, but it may only take us so far. Other factors, like addiction, can dramatically weaken willpower no matter how steadfast and devoted we think we are to a diet.

With the help of scientific research, we are beginning to understand that weight gain is closely tied to our chemistry as opposed to being an indication of our character. For example, studies have revealed that certain genes are linked to obesity, and these genes may predispose certain individuals to overeat.[2] Much as there is a genetic component to alcoholism, some people may have a genetic drive to want to eat too much of certain types of foods, and genetics can be a tough opponent for willpower. Additionally, our modern-day food environment is filled with many foods and associated stimuli that can weaken our willpower to resist them.

Just Being on a Diet Sets You Up for Failure

Another reason diets fail is because of the term *diet*. The word *diet* gets tossed around pretty casually in everyday conversation, and it is often used in different contexts. In this book, *diet* is used, for lack of a better word, to mean the food that you regularly consume and live off of. We prefer the phrase *eating plan* over *diet*, but since *diet* is used most often colloquially, for the sake of simplicity it will be used here as well.

You might wonder: what is so wrong with saying *diet*? The phrase *going on a diet* is normally used to describe what you do when you want to lose weight. The problem is that saying that you are going on a diet suggests that at some point you will go off of it. Psychologically, a diet connotes a temporary process; once you lose the weight and meet your health goals, you can go back to eating the way you used to. You just need to get through these next few weeks, or months, and then the suffering and inconvenience will be over, and a slimmer, healthier you can go back to enjoying all of the foods that you want, including those "forbidden foods" that diets typically eliminate.

Here is the bad news: this is not going to happen.

Although it isn't always obvious and they often make it look effortless, people who are thin and in good shape *don't* get to eat insane amounts of junk food and give into every food desire they have and still look that way. Maybe they indulge once in a while, but in order to stay slim, they most likely have developed an eating strategy that allows them to stay that way permanently. If you want to lose weight and keep it off, a diet needs to be a *way* of eating, not a short-term solution.

Quick Fixes Don't Work

Many diet programs out there are quick fixes: drink this mysterious liquid for seven days and you will lose fifteen pounds and end up slim and happy, just like the model in the advertisement. While that sounds like the ideal situation, the truth is, quick fixes don't last. If the lack of success with other diets you have tried is not enough to convince you, consider this: sure, you can go *on* a diet and maybe you will lose weight, but once you go *off* that diet, the weight will creep back on and you will be back to square one, sometimes with even more to lose. This cycle is evident from the rampant yo-yo dieting seen in our society, and the weight regain that is all too common among dieters. Research also shows that people who use quick-fix approaches to weight loss, such as skipping meals and taking diet pills, are actually more likely to have an increase in their body mass index (BMI, a measure used to determine whether a person is normal weight, overweight, or obese) than those who don't.[3] This underscores the futility of these quick-fix attempts. Diets, as we know them, just don't work.

It turns out that it's the opposite of the quick-fix approach that seems to do the trick when it comes to losing weight and keeping it off. Studies suggest that people who lose weight gradually are more likely to sustain their weight loss. In one study, two weight-loss approaches were compared: one that lasted twenty weeks, and another designed exactly the same but that lasted forty weeks. Weight-loss techniques were introduced to the participants in the forty-week group at a slower, more gradual pace than the twenty-week group. The results showed that individuals in the forty-week group lost more weight and were able to better maintain this weight loss over time.[4] Why? These positive effects were most likely seen because people who lost the weight slowly were making gradual changes and easing into a new way of eating, instead of adopting the quick-fix mentality that is marketed all around us.

Why does weight seem to stay off when it comes off more slowly? It may have to do with the fact that, psychologically and behaviorally, it is much easier to enact small changes over time than to try to change everything all at once. Suppose, for example, that you want to teach your dog to perform a complicated trick that contains several acts in a certain sequence—such as to climb up a steep incline, jump through a hoop, and then sit down. If you try to teach the dog all three steps at the same time, learning might never actually occur. Instead, your best bet is to reward the dog at first for simply climbing the incline, then only reward it for climbing the incline and jumping through the hoop, and finally only reward it for doing all three actions in order. It will take some time and patience, but this method will work. This approach is a psychological learning strategy known as shaping, which incorporates change slowly so that the subject can learn each step involved without becoming confused or overwhelmed.

Similarly, when we make gradual changes to our eating patterns over time, we may be more likely to develop healthy eating habits and, as a result, lose more weight than people who attempt to make drastic changes to their eating patterns overnight. So, when you jump-start yourself into a new way of eating, trying to change *all* of your bad eating behaviors at once might actually sabotage you from the start.

In order to lose weight and keep it off, long-term (lifelong) changes are needed. Although it would be great if there were a quick fix, as with much else in life, quick fixes usually only act as Band-Aids, temporarily alleviating or distracting you from the problem without actually eliminating it. For these and other reasons that will be covered next, to lose weight and maintain weight loss, you need to make a permanent change in the way that you eat, rather than going on a diet in the way that this term is typically used. Instead, diet should refer to the way you eat, now and forever. The simple truth is that you need to make a conscious decision to eat a certain way and continue to eat that way if you want to achieve and maintain weight loss—so from here on out, tell yourself that your diet is the way you eat *all of the time*, not just until you reach a fleeting milestone.

The Problem with Diets You Have Tried in the Past

How many different diets have you tried over the years? Why didn't they work for you? What were the problems with each one? At the end of the chapter, we'll ask you to make a list of the diets you've been on and note the reasons why they failed. Below are some common reasons why we abandon diet plans. We're sure that some of these issues will show up on your list.

PROBLEM #1: I'M HUNGRY!

One common problem when trying to lose weight is that we often feel hungry. This is probably one of the biggest reasons we quit a diet. The challenge when trying to lose weight is that for weight loss to occur, we need to eat less food, but as we lose weight, we actually need even fewer calories in order to maintain our new, lighter body weight. A person who weighs 125 pounds, for example, needs fewer calories to maintain that body weight (when activity and metabolic levels are controlled for) than a person who weighs 200 pounds. Essentially, the more weight you lose, the less you can eat if you want to stay that size. And if you want to continue to lose weight, you'll have to eat even fewer calories. So, if you are 200 pounds and want to lose weight, you will probably feel hungry on most diets because in order to achieve this goal you need to eat less than you are used to consuming.

Yes, you need to reduce your caloric intake to lose weight, but caloric intake does not always directly match hunger levels. Certain foods make us feel fuller, or more satiated, than others. For example, later in the book you will learn about how liquid calories (for example, sugar-sweetened beverages) are less satiating than solid foods comprised of the same number of calories. Also, the components (or ingredients) of a food can affect how much it satisfies your hunger. Similarly, certain types of food can make you feel hungry or provoke you to eat more and more of them. We will discuss this in greater detail in later chapters, but for now, keep in mind that *what* you eat is equally as important if not more important for losing weight as *how much* you eat.

PROBLEM #2: I CAN'T AFFORD TO
BUY ALL THIS FANCY FOOD!

Another barrier that you may have encountered when trying to diet is the cost of buying nutritious foods. If you go to the grocery store and look at the cost of buying a pound of fresh apples compared to a large bag of potato chips, you will probably find that the apples are more expensive. Likewise, researchers have shown that foods with a higher energy density (those that have more calories packed in each ounce of food) are less expensive than foods with a lower energy density.[5] So you can spend less money and buy more food; however, what you purchase will consist of added sugar, fat, and refined grains.[6] This means that while trying to reduce costs by buying cheaper foods, you may be contributing to the size of your waistline.

Interestingly, there is evidence demonstrating that, over time, eating a lower-calorie, nutritious diet did *not* increase diet costs.[7] In this study, families with a child between the ages of eight and twelve in an obesity treatment program participated in sessions that focused on decreasing consumption of calorie-dense foods. After one year, dietary costs were significantly *decreased*. So while it may seem that you are spending more on food as you transition from eating processed and refined foods to those that are lower in sugar, over time, the amount of money you spend on food may actually be reduced. You are making an investment in yourself and it will be a better investment overall if you eat healthy.

PROBLEM #3: I DON'T HAVE TIME TO MAKE ALL THESE MEALS!

In some ways, time and dollar costs can be a double-edged sword. Even if we save money by buying less food or not going to restaurants or fast-food chains as often, we may increase the amount of time we spend chopping, seasoning, cooking, and preparing fresh meals.[8] For many of us, time is a precious commodity. Between commuting, work meetings, spending time with friends, volunteer work, and children's soccer practices and ballet classes, the thought of adding one more thing to your metaphoric plate may seem daunting—but fear not! There are many little ways to make preparing healthy meals easy (see box on page 28).

PROBLEM #4: I DON'T HAVE THE ENERGY TO WORK OUT THIS OFTEN!

All of us have had our own unique triumphs and struggles when it comes to consistently incorporating exercise into our daily lives. Maybe in the past you have gotten bored of doing the same motions day after day and week after week or you found exercising more of a burden than an enjoyable activity. Maybe you found that it took too much energy to work out on a consistent basis, or you never seemed to find the time. Whatever the reason may be, you are not alone in how you feel.

Throughout this book, you will see that an important component of implementing this plan and changing your lifestyle is doing what is right for you. For example, the Centers for Disease Control and Prevention (CDC) has physical activity recommendations for adults, such as doing 150 minutes of moderate intensity aerobic activity (like brisk walking) every week along with muscle-strengthening activities on two or more days; or doing 75 minutes of

Tips for Preparing Healthy Meals

- Try to set aside time to decide on and plan your week's menu, perhaps with other members of your family, before going to the store. In addition to making sure that your kitchen is stocked with healthy options for the week, planning recipes ahead of time can help cut costs as common ingredients can be chosen and purchased for several different meals.

- Take just a half hour to an hour each week to precook: slice vegetables to have ready for salad toppings or side dishes, or make enough of your favorite low-carb/low-sugar meals, like crustless quiches, stews, and soups, to freeze for later in the week. In fact, whenever you cook, try to make extra that you can store and save for the next day.

- As with almost everything else in life, your attitude toward cooking can make all the difference. Instead of treating it as a source of stress or a time-consuming task, try to view cooking as enjoyable and even calming! Preparing a meal can be an opportunity to wind down after a long day or a fun activity for the whole family.

jogging, running, or other vigorous intensity aerobic activity along with muscle-strengthening activities on two or more days. You can break the activities into ten-minute chunks of time.[9] The CDC also recommends scheduling your workouts at the times during the day or week when you have energy.[10] If you are someone who feels energetic in the morning, then try working out before you go to work. If you prefer the middle of the day, try going for a brisk walk during your lunch hour, maybe with a friend. If you are a night owl, work out while you watch television after you get home. Regardless of the time of day or activities that you prefer, find what works for you and feel free to make adjustments as you go. The key is to make sure that you consistently elevate your heart rate and stay committed.

Changing your eating habits can help you lose weight, but you must also stay active to tone your muscles.

PROBLEM #5: I DON'T KNOW WHICH DIET WILL WORK!

There are tons of programs, pills, shakes, juices, and books out there to help you lose weight—so many, in fact, that it can be hard to decide which ones might actually be worth trying. Over the past twenty years, we have seen our fair share of diet fads. The Beverly Hills Diet, the Grapefruit Diet, the Cabbage Soup Diet, the Baby Food Diet, and liquid fasts—this is just a handful of the many fad diets that have been developed and tried over the years. It may seem as though once you've learned all that is involved in one approach, another diet comes on the market with an entirely different focus, leaving you to wonder which types of food are really important to reduce in your diet and which should be included for your health and weight-loss goals. In the 1990s, we were told by the U.S. Food and Drug Administration (FDA) to reduce fat intake. That was the start of the low-fat diet revolution. High-carbohydrate diets were readily available; people all over were cutting back on hamburgers and bacon, and eating anything and everything that was "fat-free." Certainly, cutting out excess amounts of fat can reduce calorie intake, but the problem was the calories that previously came from fat were often replaced by calories from bread, pasta, pretzels, and "fat-free" diet foods. Although many people joined the fat-free diet revolution, as a society, our body weights continued to increase. The fat-free diet just didn't seem to work well to sustain long-term weight loss.

In more recent years, the tables have turned: fat has become less demonized, and research suggests that weight-loss efforts may be more successful if they are aimed at reducing carbohydrate intake. Excessive intake of carbohydrates is a source of excess calories and body weight, and surveys suggest that most people eat more carbohydrates than they think they should.[11] There is science to back the idea that low-carbohydrate diets can work. A study featured in the *New England Journal of Medicine* showed that both a low-carbohydrate diet and a Mediterranean-style diet (which is also low in carbohydrates) are significantly more effective in reducing body weight compared to a low-fat diet.[12] Likewise, another study found that a diet allowing only limited carbohydrate intake was more effective in producing short-term weight loss among women who were obese than a low-fat diet with a focus on limited caloric intake.[13]

PROBLEM #6: LOW-CARBOHYDRATE DIETS ARE HARD TO STICK TO

So, if a low-carbohydrate diet seems to be the best bet for sustained weight loss, why isn't everyone on one and losing weight? Herein lies the problem: what is good isn't always easy. In one survey, 87 percent of respondents reported that they crave carbohydrates (like bread, pasta, and rice) about eleven times per week, suggesting the large role that they play in the diet of many people.[14] Given this finding, it is no surprise that a big problem with low-carbohydrate diets is that people seem to have a lot of difficulty staying on them.

Sticking to a low-carb diet is often hard because of "carb confusion." There are several different low-carbohydrate diets out there, and different ways of counting carbohydrates. There are lots of different terms, like *net carbs*, *good carbs*, *bad carbs*, and *glycemic index*, which can be confusing, complicated, and sometimes even contradictory as you try to decide which foods to eat. Also, some low-carb diets are very restrictive, while others seem more relaxed. Deciding which foods are acceptable and which are not can be hard. A survey suggests that most people consider vegetables and whole grains to be healthy carbs, but many people also think that fruit juices and jams or jellies are good carbohydrates to consume; however, as it turns out, fruit juices, jams, and jellies are *not* healthy carbs, as they often contain high amounts of added sugar.[15] One of the key reasons low-carb diets fail, which has been ignored up until this point, is *addiction* to carbohydrate-rich foods, which might be making adherence to low-carbohydrate diets difficult. In this book, we will simplify the carbohydrate conundrum and explain how you can eat a low-carbohydrate diet in a way that is easy to understand.

✳

Understanding why diets typically fail can help you be more successful with changing your eating habits in the future. Knowing what you can—and can't—control and recognizing why certain diets may not have worked for you in the past will help you to focus your efforts for the best results.

In the next chapter, we'll help you take stock of your current sugar intake so you can start reducing it. It's probably much higher than you think—and easier to cut down on than you might expect.

FOOD FOR THOUGHT

List five of the different diet approaches you have tried in the past. Then consider each.

- What about each plan didn't work for you?
- Do you notice a common theme?

By knowing which aspects of your previous dieting attempts may have contributed to their failure, you become aware of your weaknesses. You may also identify areas over which you don't have much control, such as feeling like you have an addiction to sugary drinks or carbohydrate-rich pasta dishes.

STEP 2

Weigh In on Your Sugar Intake

"A bagel is a doughnut with the sin removed."

—GEORGE ROSENBAUM, FOOD-INDUSTRY ANALYST

The FDA has a long history of issuing governmental dietary recommendations, beginning all the way back in 1894, to help us know which foods we should eat and how we should structure our diets. The idea is to provide simple, useful information for individuals to employ in their everyday lives and food-intake decisions. Foods can be divided into three general categories to describe their contents: carbohydrates, fats, and protein. Most of us recall that, back in the 1990s, the FDA introduced the food pyramid, which emphasized that the majority of our food intake should come from carbohydrates, such as breads and pasta, with fats consumed very sparingly. Then in 2005, the FDA revised the food pyramid to reflect slightly less emphasis on whole grains and other carbohydrates (although these still dominated as the major food group). It also recommended exercise and acknowledged that age, gender, and activity levels are all factors to be considered when determining healthy food-intake patterns.

Today the guidelines have been completely revamped, and we no longer follow a pyramid model. Instead, we have the food plate model,[1] which suggests that half of our plate be filled with fruits and vegetables. Whole fruits and fruit juices are recommended. Grains (another type of carbohydrate) are recommended to comprise approximately one-quarter of our plate, and the same goes for protein. We are also advised to have a small portion of dairy products.

The food plate guidelines also caution people to avoid "empty calories." Empty calories are often found in foods that contain sugars and solid fats, which are added to foods to make them more appealing. These calories are considered "empty" because they offer few or no nutrients; they are just calories that need to be burned or they will turn into excess body weight. What's the biggest culprit in terms of empty calories in our food today? Sodas, which are sweetened with sugars like sucrose or high-fructose corn syrup.

What is interesting about empty calories is their appeal. These foods taste really, really good, and thus people want to eat lots of them. But they are not necessary for survival, so eating them excessively or in place of nutrient-rich foods does not make sense. This preference for foods that are highly palatable but lacking in nutritive value may form the foundation for what can develop into an addiction. If this is the case, trying to avoid eating them or attempting to eat them in moderation might be easier said than done.

The bottom line is that governmental food guidelines have shifted over the years, in part to incorporate developments in nutrition research and perhaps after recognizing that too many sugars and other carbohydrates are not ideal for a healthy body weight. We say "sugar and *other carbohydrates*" here because, technically,

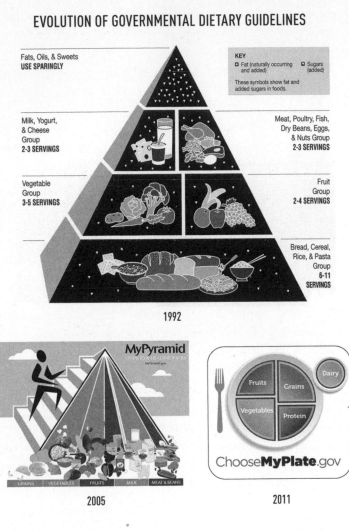

EVOLUTION OF GOVERNMENTAL DIETARY GUIDELINES

Fats, Oils, & Sweets
USE SPARINGLY

KEY
☐ Fat (naturally occurring and added)   ☐ Sugars (added)

These symbols show fat and added sugars in foods.

Milk, Yogurt, & Cheese Group
2-3 SERVINGS

Meat, Poultry, Fish, Dry Beans, Eggs, & Nuts Group
2-3 SERVINGS

Vegetable Group
3-5 SERVINGS

Fruit Group
2-4 SERVINGS

Bread, Cereal, Rice, & Pasta Group
6-11 SERVINGS

1992

MyPyramid
STEPS TO A HEALTHIER YOU
MyPyramid.gov

GRAINS   VEGETABLES   FRUITS   MILK   MEAT & BEANS

2005

Fruits   Grains   Dairy
Vegetables   Protein

ChooseMyPlate.gov

2011

Adapted from USDA Center For Nutrition Policy and Promotion (2011). A brief history of USDA food guides. Retrieved from http://www.choosemyplate .gov/foodgroups/downloads/MyPlate/ABriefHistoryOfUSDAFoodGuides.pdf. Accessed on August 14, 2012.

sugar is a general term used to describe what is really a carbohydrate. When most people refer to sugar, however, they are probably talking about table sugar—the white stuff you put in your coffee or use to whip up a batch of cookies—which is technically called *sucrose*. It's important to understand the difference between foods (like complex carbohydrates) that break down into biochemical sugars and the more common table sugar (sucrose) because you'll need to reduce or cut out both of these types of sugars in order to end your addiction. As we've said (and will cover in more detail in Step 4), both clinical testimony and scientific support suggests that some people who overeat sugars and other carbohydrates may have an addiction to them, and this addiction may explain why adhering to a low-carbohydrate diet and achieving a sustained weight loss can be such a challenge. So what is the connection between sugar, carbohydrates, and weight loss?

Breaking Down Carbohydrates

Carbohydrates can be complex, not only in their form but also when trying to understand all of the jargon that is used to describe them. In simplest terms, when talking about diet, a carbohydrate is a source of energy (for instance, calories) that includes things we commonly know as sugars and starches. This isn't going to be a biochemistry lesson, but it is important to cover some of the basics regarding carbohydrate metabolism, as this background information will be important for you to keep in mind as you start to think about the kinds of foods you like to eat and the addiction-like behaviors that might be leading you to overeat.

SIMPLE VERSUS COMPLEX CARBOHYDRATES

You are probably already familiar with some of the many terms associated with carbohydrates. In general, when carbohydrates are discussed, they are referred to as *simple carbohydrates* such as sucrose, high-fructose corn syrup, and glucose, or as *complex carbohydrates* that make up things like breads and pastas. This division into simple and complex is not exactly a perfect model for understanding the nutritional value of carbohydrates. Complex carbohydrates such as brown rice and many vegetables are often viewed as healthy carbohydrates, while simple carbohydrates such as table sugar and fruit sugar are less healthy. However, some complex carbohydrates, like french fries, are certainly not healthy, and some simple carbohydrates, like whole fruits, are an important part of your diet because they contain other important nutrients and fiber.

So what is the difference between simple and complex carbohydrates, and why does it matter? It turns out that there are key differences in the way that simple and complex carbohydrates are processed and broken down to be utilized by our bodies, which can affect the way that eating them makes us feel.

As we digest our food, our bodies break down all carbohydrates (both simple and complex) and obtain, among other nutrients, glucose. *Glucose* is the energy that is essential for life. It is the fuel for our cells and is used throughout our bodies. Some glucose is used immediately as energy. If it is not used immediately, our bodies store glucose in a different form, called *glycogen*. When we need extra energy, like when we rigorously exercise, our bodies can use the glycogen stockpiles and turn them into energy.

Simple carbohydrates are more easily and readily broken down by our bodies because their chemical structure is rather "simple"— it is made up of just one or two sugar molecules linked together. Simple carbohydrates break down in our bodies right away, and as a result they cause immediate increases in blood sugar levels. This is why simple carbohydrates are sometimes referred to as *fast carbohydrates*. Conversely, complex carbohydrates contain three or more sugar molecules. As a result, our bodies take a longer time to digest them, and they don't raise sugar levels in the blood as quickly as simple carbohydrates. This is why they are often referred to as *slow carbohydrates*.

THE GLYCEMIC INDEX

Many people find it more useful to think about simple versus complex carbohydrates in the way that they influence our blood sugar levels. Slow carbohydrates (complex carbohydrates) raise your blood sugar levels at a gradual pace and give your body a steady stream of fuel. Brown rice, lentils, oatmeal, whole wheat bread, vegetables, and fiber-rich fruits are examples of slow carbohydrates.

Fast carbohydrates (simple carbohydrates), on the other hand, enter your bloodstream at a fast pace and cause your blood sugar to spike and dip, which causes your body to produce large amounts of a hormone called *insulin*. Insulin is needed to turn the sugar in your blood into a usable sugar that can enter your cells. Insulin helps to convert blood sugar into energy or stores it for later use in other places (such as your liver or muscles). If you have too much excess blood sugar floating around, insulin can even convert it into fat stores. Eating a lot of fast carbohydrates such as white bread, donuts, and soda can increase your chances of having energy dips, becoming irritable, and getting hungry quickly between meals. These feelings are also associated with the withdrawal you feel when you go for periods of time without eating these foods.

A system known as the *glycemic index* helps classify carbohydrates based on how quickly they increase your blood sugar and to what level. Fast carbohydrates are on the high end of the glycemic index and slow carbohydrates are on the low end. Some studies suggest that a diet rich in high-glycemic-index foods, which cause blood sugar to spike and dip faster than low-glycemic-index foods, may increase your likelihood of overeating[2] and may be linked to heart disease[3] and diabetes.[4]

✳

What does all of this mean? Based on what we've described so far, you would be right to assume that you should eat some carbohydrates as part of a healthy diet, but avoid ones that have empty calories and are fast digesting, as these can lead to you to overeat and then, shortly afterward, feel hungry and irritable. Here is the problem: those fast-digesting carbs made up of empty calories are delicious, and many of us *love* to eat these types of foods. Cutting back on our intake of these carbohydrates can be difficult not only because they are tasty but also because they are cheap, convenient, and readily available. And there is a biological basis for the desire to eat these types of carbohydrates, sugars in particular, which may lead you to become addicted to them and thus hinder efforts to remain on a low-carbohydrate diet. We have an evolutionary tendency to view things that are sweet as being safe. For example, if our ancestors were to come upon a berry patch in the wild, those berries that were ripe and safe berries would taste sweet, whereas rotten ones would not.

Luckily, it is possible to overcome these challenges and cut back on your intake of fast-digesting carbs with empty calories. Understanding why these carbs end up being stored as fat is the first step. In Step 4, we'll help you begin to reduce these carbs until, at the end of the book, you will have cut them out completely!

The Many Faces of Sugar

Sometimes it can be difficult to understand which foods are actually sugars. Contrary to what we normally think of when we envision a sugar, not all sugars taste very sweet and not all things that are sweet (for example, artificial sweeteners and sugar substitutes) are considered sugars.

As you can see from the box on page 40, there are lots of different sugars and sweeteners out there. While sugars like those on this list are grouped into the same class for the purposes of this book, it is important to underscore that they are not exactly the same. Aside from the obvious differences that some are sweet and some are not and that they are derived from various sources (for example, corn sugar comes from a different source than beet sugar), scientists continue to uncover other intrinsic differences among various types of sweeteners and their effects on the body.

WHERE ARE SUGARS?

As mentioned earlier, our bodies need to make glucose (a sugar) to survive, so sugar plays an important role in our diet and health. However, this does not mean that you need to *eat* sugars to get glucose; your body can break down fats and proteins to make glucose when needed as well.

Most of us eat more sugar than we need, and often this sugar is consumed blindly. We don't always realize how much sugar is actually in the foods we eat, and foods that contain empty calories are not clearly marked. While we often see food items that are labeled "low-fat" or "fat-free," we never see a food labeled "nonnutritious" or "junk food."

The labels are there, but it is up to the consumer to know how to read them. So, in order for you to properly evaluate the amount of sugars contained in a given food, it's important to understand how to interpret a nutrition label. These labels are often on the back of food packages, but sometimes, as in the case of chain or fast-food restaurants, this information is not readily available, and you may need to request it (or you can usually find it on the company's website). An example of a typical nutrition label is shown on page 42; this one is for a package of Skittles candy.

There have been efforts put forth recently to make calorie content and nutrition information more visible to people, in the hopes that providing such information will enable us to make more

A Sugar by Any Other Name . . .

Agave nectar	Florida crystals	Maltodextrin
Barbados sugar	Free-flowing brown	Maltose
Barley malt	sugar	Mannitol
Beet sugar	Fructose	Maple syrup
Blackstrap molasses	Fruit juice	Molasses
Brown sugar	Fruit juice concentrate	Muscovado sugar
Cane crystals	Galactose	Organic raw sugar
Cane juice crystals	Glucose	Panocha
Cane sugar	Glucose solids	Powdered sugar
Caramel	Golden sugar	Raw sugar
Carob syrup	Golden syrup	Refiner's syrup
Castor sugar	Granulated sugar	Rice syrup
Confectioner's sugar	Grape juice concentrate	Sorbitol
Corn sweetener	Grape sugar	Sorghum syrup
Corn syrup	HFCS	Sucrose
Corn syrup solids	High-fructose corn	Sugar
Crystalline fructose	syrup	Table sugar
Date sugar	Honey	Treacle
Demerara sugar	Icing sugar	Turbinado sugar
Dextrose	Invert sugar	Yellow sugar
D-mannose	Lactose	
Evaporated cane juice	Malt syrup	

informed food choices. Has making this information more accessible worked? Unfortunately, it hasn't. And this has nothing to do with intelligence or comprehension levels; adults with low levels of literacy and numeracy and those with higher levels of education have both been shown to have difficulty understanding nutrition labels.[5]

Part of the problem is that these labels are meaningless if we don't understand how to interpret them. Also, as you will soon see, the way that the information is presented on the labels can be misleading. So, let's dissect a label piece by piece so you can understand what all of this information means.

PERCENT DAILY VALUE (%DV)

The upper right of the label reads "%DV*," meaning the percent daily value based on a 2,000-calorie-per-day diet. In essence, the numbers that are listed under this heading indicate how much a serving of that food contributes to the overall recommended daily intake of a particular category, whether the category is total fat, total carbohydrates, or a certain vitamin. For example, the label above shows that one serving of this item contributes 13 percent of the recommended daily intake of saturated fat that is suggested by the FDA.

In addition to the %DV, the nutrition facts also tell you how many grams of fat, cholesterol, sodium, total carbohydrates, and protein are found in one serving size of the item. This label indicates, for instance, that one serving of Skittles contains 56 grams of carbohydrates, 47 of which are sugar. These two items, the number of grams of carbohydrates and the number of grams of sugar that come from carbohydrates, are both important when trying to determine if a certain food fits with your goal to reduce your sugar and carbohydrate intake. However, to make food-intake decisions easily

```
Nutrition Facts
Serving Size (61.5g)
Calories 250
```

Amount/Serving	%DV*
Total Fat 2.5g	4%
Saturated Fat 2.5g	13%
Trans Fat 0g	
Cholesterol 0mg	0%
Sodium 10mg	0%
Total Carbohydrate 56g	19%
Dietary Fiber 0g	0%
Sugars 47g	
Protein 0g	

* Percent Daily Values (DV) are based on a 2,000 calorie diet.

INGREDIENTS: SUGAR, CORN SYRUP, HYDROGENATED PALM KERNEL OIL, APPLE JUICE FROM CONCENTRATE, LESS THAN 2% CITRIC ACID, DEXTRIN, MODIFIED CORN STARCH, NATURAL AND ARTIFICIAL FLAVORS, COLORING (INCLUDES YELLOW 6 LAKE, RED 40 LAKE, YELLOW 5 LAKE, BLUE 2 LAKE, YELLOW 5, RED 40, YELLOW 6, BLUE 1 LAKE, BLUE 1), ASCORBIC ACID (VITAMIN C).

Adapted from www.wrigley.com/global/brands/skittles.aspx#panel-3. Accessed on August 14, 2012.

(and without a calculator), we've compiled the Sugar Equivalency Table for you (see page 195), which will help you easily identify how much sugar is contained in a food and whether or not that food fits with your diet plan. We will explain in greater detail how to interpret and use this table in upcoming chapters.

SERVING SIZE

When using nutrition labels, determining the appropriate serving size can also be a tricky thing. Just glancing at a nutrition label can be misleading and dangerous. If you down an entire package of cookies thinking it is one serving, and it turns out the package contained four servings, then you just consumed quadruple the number of calories, carbohydrates, and sugars you thought you did. Some labels will tell you how many servings are in the entire package. Others will tell you how many pieces are in a serving size. This package tells you one serving is 61.5 grams. Do you know off the top of your head how many Skittles would equal a 61.5 gram serving? (In case you're wondering, it's approximately sixty-two Skittles.) Most people don't walk around with scales and weigh out every morsel of food before they eat it. The point is that nutrition labels aren't always very user-friendly, and you often have to do some quick math in your head in order to get a realistic assessment of how much of something you're actually eating.

INGREDIENTS LIST

Below the nutritional information on a label is a list of ingredients. Importantly, these ingredients are listed in order of the amount contained in the product, with the ingredients contained in larger amounts listed first. In this example, you can see that sugar is the primary ingredient in Skittles. Sugar is often one of the first few ingredients listed on the nutrition label. If the word *sugar* isn't there, in its place might be another one of the many terms used to describe different types of sugars (see the box on page 40), such as high-fructose corn syrup, corn syrup, fruit juice concentrate, maltose, and dextrose. All of these terms can be confusing and difficult to remember. However, an article published in the *Journal of the*

American Dietetic Association offers some helpful tips for determining whether added sugars are contained in a food or beverage (see sidebar). Also note that "sugar" can appear more than once in the list of ingredients. For example, on the Skittles label, you actually get "sugar" from the majority of the ingredients (sugar, corn syrup, apple juice from concentrate, dextrin, and modified corn starch).

How to Identify Added Sugars[6]

- Search the ingredient list for the word *syrup*, such as corn syrup, high-fructose corn syrup, maple syrup, and agave syrup.

- Look for words ending in "ose," such as fructose, glucose, sucrose, and dextrose.

- Compare the unsweetened version of a product (plain, unsweetened yogurt or plain shredded wheat cereal) with the sweetened version (fruit-flavored yogurt or frosted shredded wheat) to estimate the amount of added sugars.

- Beware of a "health halo" effect. Some added sugars, such as brown rice syrup, may sound healthful but they are just other forms of added sweeteners.

2,000-CALORIE DIET

It's important to note that these nutritional guidelines are pretty generic; they are the same for a third-grader as they are for a high school football player and a middle-aged businesswoman. In reality, however, each person is different and has different daily nutritional needs depending on a wide variety of factors, including age, activity level, preexisting health conditions, and so on. Further, not everyone needs 2,000 calories per day to maintain their body weight; some may need more, while others need less. One label cannot possibly indicate the diverse caloric and nutritional needs of so many different-ent people. Rather, nutritional labels are meant to serve as an average or a guide. While it is important to interpret nutrition labels with caution and to understand that they are not tailored specifically to our individual nutritional needs, nutrition labels do provide us with essential information about the ingredients and nutrients in the foods we eat, which can be especially helpful to consider when trying to cut down on the consumption of certain ingredients in particular.

All You *Can* Eat, or All You *Should* Eat?

The discussion of serving sizes brings up another important point to consider when evaluating any diet: portion sizes. Since the 1970s, the portion size of many foods and beverages has increased, not only in our favorite fast-food establishments but also at other restaurants, in schools, and at home.[7, 8] This increase in portion sizes parallels the increases in our waist sizes during this time period, and studies suggest that this isn't a coincidence. When we're provided with larger portions, we tend to eat more.[9] All-you-can-eat buffet? Let's not even go there—literally!

Many of us have come to consider what is placed in front of us, or in the package that we purchase, as the amount we're supposed to eat. When we go to a restaurant and the waiter places a plate of food in front of us, most of us eat what is on the plate even though it is much more food than what we might normally eat in a given meal. Further, people state that they base how much they eat on the amount that they are used to eating.[10, 11] If people eat based on previous experiences, and portion sizes are larger than necessary or healthy, then it is no wonder so many people are overweight. Basing our food intake on social norms or the amount considered appropriate by a restaurant or fast-food chain is a recipe for disaster.

In later chapters when we discuss the criteria for addiction, you'll learn about the concept of *tolerance*. Most people are already familiar with this term and know that part of an addiction involves becoming tolerant to the substance of abuse, and tolerance for addictive substances increases over time. This means that, over time, we have to consume more of the substance to satisfy our addiction. If sugar-rich and high-carbohydrate foods are potentially addictive, this means that people might need to consume larger and more frequent portions in order to satisfy their "hunger," which is really not hunger but their addiction.

How does this relate to portion sizes? Well, this is exactly what we have seen happening in the marketplace. Fifty years ago, people ate chocolate candies that they purchased for one penny out of a jar at the neighborhood store. Then candy bars came into existence, but each was typically rather small, if you can remember the size of the original Hershey's or Milky Way bar. Since then, candy bars have grown enormously in size. In fact, now you can buy Hershey bars that are more than three times larger than the original size. Consumer demand is what drives the market.

Similarly, over time, sugary sodas have gotten much larger. In the 1930s a typical Coca-Cola bottle, for example, was just 6 ounces, but now the standard-size can is 12-ounces. And now sodas are available in 32-ounce, 48-ounce, and even 64-ounce sizes. Car companies had to start making larger cup holders in cars to accommodate such beverages. We see the same thing when we look at the ice-cream treats in the convenience-store freezer. Ice cream started in very small Dixie cups solely in the vanilla flavor. Over time, ice-cream manufacturers added much greater sugar content by adding chocolate sauces and sugary fruit toppings. The invention of the ice-cream sandwich added chocolate wafers to the mixture. Recently, we have

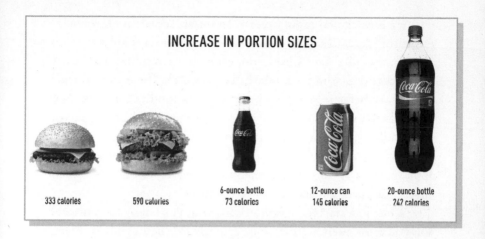

INCREASE IN PORTION SIZES

		6-ounce bottle	12-ounce can	20-ounce bottle
333 calories	590 calories	73 calories	145 calories	242 calories

seen ice-cream sandwiches explode in size and now include huge chocolate chip cookies to hold them together rather than chocolate wafers. Knowing how to read nutrition labels to determine serving size and recognizing that portion sizes have grown dramatically in recent years will help you figure out how much sugar you are actually consuming.

How Much Sugar Are You Really Eating?

The table on page 49 illustrates the sugar content in some popular foods to give you an idea of how much sugar you may be taking in. When looking at this table, you may begin to realize that you consume much more sugar than you imagined, and certainly more than you need. You might also notice that certain foods and beverages that appear harmless or even healthy actually contain very high amounts of sugar. A bottle of Peach Snapple Iced Tea, for example, contains just as many grams of sugar as a can of Coca-Cola!

With work and family responsibilities, social commitments, and leisure activities, little time is left over these days for preparing meals and snacks. For this reason, processed foods and drinks are extremely popular in the modern Western diet. These convenience foods have become a staple in our modern food culture, as they enable us to quickly and easily satisfy our hunger while we engage in the daily grind of our fast-paced lifestyles. These processed foods and drinks are convenient because they rarely require refrigeration, don't spoil easily, and often come in cans, boxes, or cartons, which make transportation and storage convenient.

When you start to look more closely at your daily food intake, you will most likely see that you regularly eat these types of foods, and perhaps more than you thought. And you're not alone—research shows that people, in general, value convenience a lot. We consume more and more foods from fast-food and full-service restaurants, many of which are heavily processed and laden with excess sugars and fats. In fact, research shows that between 1977 and 1978, 16 percent of people's meals came from places outside the home. By 1995, this number had increased to approximately 29 percent.[12] When you add in the amount of processed and prepackaged foods that we consume *inside* of the home, this number goes up even higher. When we take a step back and consider our own eating patterns and the research regarding the eating patterns of others, it is clear that, unfortunately, we often value convenience over nutrition, and most of us are probably not even aware that we're making this tradeoff.

When thinking about such "convenience" foods, a theme emerges: these foods are loaded with sugars. It might surprise you that sugar is not only found in the sodas and condiments offered at fast-food restaurants but also in foods that appear healthy, like some granola bars.

SUGAR CONTENT IN POPULAR FOODS

FOOD OR BEVERAGE ITEM	TOTAL SUGARS (G)	TOTAL CALORIES	CALORIES FROM SUGAR	% OF CALORIES FROM SUGAR
Bertolli Vineyard Marinara Sauce (1/2 cup)	12	90	48	53%
Chobani Greek Yogurt, Nonfat, Raspberry (1 cup)	19	140	76	54%
Coca-Cola (12 fl. oz.)	39	140	140	100%
Craisins (1/4 cup)	29	130	116	89%
Dole Diced Peaches in 100% Fruit Juice (1/2 cup)	18	80	72	90%
Florida's Natural Orange Juice, Most Pulp (8 fl. oz.)	22	110	88	80%
Frosted Cherry Pop-Tart (1 pastry)	16	200	64	32%
Glaceau Vitamin Water Power-C, Dragonfruit (20 fl. oz.)	32	120	120	100%
Go-Gurt (1 tube)	10	70	40	57%
Jell-O Fat-free 100-Calorie Pudding Snack, Chocolate Vanilla Swirl (110g)	16	100	64	64%
Mott's Apple Juice (8 fl. oz.)	28	120	112	93%
Mott's Apple Sauce, Original (1 cup)	22	90	88	97%
POM Pomegranate Juice (8 fl. oz.)	32	150	128	85%
Power Bar, Peanut Butter (1 bar)	26	240	104	43%
Snapple Peach Iced Tea (16 fl. oz.)	39	160	156	97%
Sweet Baby Ray's Honey BBQ Sauce (2 tablespoons)	15	70	60	85%
V8 Fusion Vegetable Fruit, Peach Mango (8 fl. oz.)	26	120	104	86%
Weight Watchers Mint Chocolate Chip Ice Cream Cup (1 cup)	19	140	76	54%
Yoplait Yogurt, Strawberry (6 oz.)	26	170	104	61%

Sugar from Fruit

Fruit contains naturally occurring sugar in several forms, including fructose, which is different from the commercially developed sweetener high-fructose corn syrup. Does this mean that you should lump fruit into the same category as other sugar-rich foods? Not necessarily. We'll discuss this topic in greater detail in part two of the book, but, for now, keep in mind that one thing that makes whole fruits (as opposed to fruit juices) different is that they are not empty calories, but rather, they contain nutrients and, more importantly, fiber. Fiber does a few different things that are beneficial to our health. *Insoluble fiber* is the type of fiber that helps move material through the digestive tract, alleviating constipation. Whole wheat flour, wheat bran, nuts, and some vegetables are good examples of sources of insoluble fiber. The type of fiber found in fruits, like apples, is *soluble fiber*, which means that it dissolves in water. Soluble fiber can help lower blood cholesterol and glucose levels and even reduce the risk of developing type 2 diabetes, as well as reduce blood pressure and inflammation. It can be found in things like oats, peas, beans, citrus fruits, carrots, and barley.

An added bonus of high-fiber foods is that they can assist in weight loss. Generally, foods that contain a lot of fiber require more chewing time, which gives your body more time to register when you're no longer hungry, so you're less likely to overeat. Also, a high-fiber diet tends to make a meal feel larger and linger longer, so you stay full for a longer period of time. High-fiber diets also tend to be less "energy dense," which means that they have fewer calories for the same volume of food. This is one key reason why, if you're trying to lose weight, you should avoid eating refined or processed foods such as canned fruits, dried fruits (which often contain added sugar), most fruit juices, white bread and pasta, and non–whole grain cereals—these foods are lower in fiber content. The grain-refining process removes the outer coat (bran) from the grain, which lowers its fiber content. Similarly, removing the skin from fruit decreases its fiber content.

So, although you may not tend to eat a lot of the typical foods, such as pastries and cookies, that often come to mind when thinking of high-sugar foods, when you add up the sugar content in processed foods, you probably consume much more sugar than you intended. From your bowl of cereal at breakfast to the pasta and soft drink you have for lunch to the ice cream you eat to satisfy your sweet tooth after dinner, sugar is omnipresent in Western diets. Let's take a look at some examples of what people might eat in a typical day (see pages 52–3). You may find that you can relate to one of them or know someone who can.

Note that the values in the table represent sugar; carbohydrates aren't included. How much sugar is considered a healthy amount? It's hard to tell bacause there aren't recommended daily intake values. The American Heart Association has guidelines for added sugar; however, no more than approximately six teaspoons for women and nine teaspoons for men.

∗

So, to recap some of the main points we have discussed so far: (1) we as a society are getting fatter and unhealthier, largely because we eat too much, (2) many of our diet attempts end in failure despite our initial motivation, (3) many of our foods contain high amounts of sugars, and we might not even be aware of this when we eat them. Is it possible that there is something about sugar in particular that may connect these three observations? Yes, sugars taste good and are therefore naturally rewarding, but sometimes we feel compelled to eat foods that contain them, even to the point where we feel a loss of control over eating. When we consider all of these points together, we face the question: is it possible that sugars could be addictive?

SUGAR INTAKE FOR FIVE DIFFERENT PEOPLE

	BREAKFAST	SNACK	LUNCH
Working Mom	• Large Dunkin' Donuts frozen coffee coolatta w/skim milk (98g) • Quaker instant oatmeal, golden brown sugar (18g) *116 grams*	None	• Chick-fil-A chicken sandwich (5g) • 2 packets ketchup (12g) • 20 oz. Coke (65g) *82 grams*
Dad with a Long Commute	• 7-Eleven sausage biscuit (2g) • Krispy Kreme old-fashioned honey and oat donut (25g) • Krispy Kreme raspberry frozen beverage (65g) *92 grams*	• 1 orange (12g) *12 grams*	• Wendy's 10-piece chicken nuggets (0g) • Sweet-and-sour nugget sauce (10g) • Large chili (8g) • Small lemonade (46g) *64 grams*
Someone Who Thinks They Are Eating Well	• Dannon fruit on the bottom 99% fat-free peach yogurt (26g) • Banana (14g) • 8 oz.Tropicana orange juice w/lots of pulp (22g) *62 grams*	None	• Panera fuji apple chicken salad (21g) • 20 oz. Lipton 100% natural iced tea w/lemon (33g) *54 grams*
10-Year-Old Child	• 2 S'mores Pop-Tart pastries (38g) • 8 oz. Minute Maid orange juice (24g) *62 grams*	None	• 2 tbsp. Skippy smooth peanut butter (3g) and 1 tbsp. Smucker's strawberry jelly (12g) • 2 slices whole wheat bread (4g) • Hi-C juice box, wild cherry (27g) *46 grams*
Recently Unemployed Person Living on a Tight Budget	Skipped	None	• Burger King premium Alaskan fish sandwich (8g) • Medium onion rings (5g) • 20 oz. Coke (65g) *78 grams*

Note: Nutritional information taken from company and nutrition information websites.

SNACK	DINNER	DESSERT/LATE-NIGHT SNACK	TOTAL GRAMS OF SUGAR PER DAY
• 3 Musketeers bar (40g) • Large Dunkin' Donuts frozen coffee coolatta w/ skim milk (98g) *134 grams*	• 56g Barilla angel hair pasta (2g) • 1/2 cup Newman's Own tomato and basil pasta sauce (9g) • 8 oz. Simply lemonade (28g) *39 grams*	• 1.69 oz. M&M's, milk chocolate (30g) *30 grams*	401 grams
• 1 Milky Way bar (35g) • 12 oz. Vanilla Coke (42g) *77 grams*	• 1/5 of a DiGiorno microwave pizza (3g) • 12 oz. A&W root beer (45g) *48 grams*	• 1 pork eggroll (5g) • 1 cup Uncle Ben's white rice (0g) *5 grams*	298 grams
• Kind walnut and date bar (16g) *16 grams*	• Smart Ones teriyaki chicken and vegetables (16g) *16 grams*	• Skinny Cow vanilla caramel cone (17g) *17 grams*	165 grams
• Entenmann's little bites blueberry muffins (14g) *14 grams*	• 1 cup Kraft macaroni and cheese (6g) • 14 oz. Nesquick low-fat chocolate milk (56g) *62 grams*	• 3 Oreos (14g) • 8 oz. whole milk (11g) *25 grams*	209 grams
• 8 oz. 7-Eleven mango medley slurpee (18g) *18 grams*	• Nathan's Brand corn dog on a stick (13g) • 20 oz. Coke (65g) *78 grams*	None	174 grams

Considering that, in some forms, sugar is a natural ingredient, and that sugars are commonly seen in our foods and drinks, it may be hard to believe that sugars could be addictive. However, as you will see in the next few chapters, the pervasiveness and excessive use of many processed and unhealthy foods, which are often rich in sugars, may have hijacked primitive brain systems that evolved to make us naturally like to eat food since we need it to survive. As a result, some of us may be faced with an unhealthy attachment to or dependence on food and a desire to overeat certain foods, which, over time, can add unwanted inches to our waistlines.

Sample Food Diary

Keeping a food diary is one way to make an honest assessment of what you eat so you can see where to make adjustments in your diet. It is also useful because it may reveal times that you are eating for reasons that aren't hunger driven. Below is an example of the type of information that you should record.

TIME	FOOD/DRINK CONSUMED	HOW MUCH?	WHY DID I EAT IT?	TOTAL SUGAR
7:30 a.m.	Brown sugar cinnamon Pop-Tarts	1 package (2 tarts)	Hungry for breakfast—on way to work	30g
1 p.m.	Frontega chicken panini on focaccia bread from Panera Bread	1 sandwich	Out to lunch with people from work	7g
4 p.m.	Coke and Reese's peanut butter cups	1 12 oz. can 1 package	Felt myself fading	39g + 21g= 60g
7 p.m.	Stouffer's mac and cheese	1 package	Dinner	8g
9:30 p.m.	Oreo cookies	3 cookies	Craving something sweet	14g

Fill-In Food Diary

Using the worksheet below, keep track of everything you eat and drink for the next five days. In the right-hand column, list the total number of sugars as well as the total number of carbohydrates in grams contained in each food item or beverage. You can do this as you go along or at the end of the five days by researching these values online. Remember to pay attention to the serving sizes listed on the package.

TIME	FOOD/DRINK CONSUMED	HOW MUCH?	WHY DID I EAT IT?	TOTAL SUGAR
DAY 1				
			TOTAL	

DAY 2				
			TOTAL	

Fill-In Food Diary, continued

TIME	FOOD/DRINK CONSUMED	HOW MUCH?	WHY DID I EAT IT?	TOTAL SUGAR
DAY 3				
			TOTAL	

TIME	FOOD/DRINK CONSUMED	HOW MUCH?	WHY DID I EAT IT?	TOTAL SUGAR
DAY 4				
			TOTAL	

TIME	FOOD/DRINK CONSUMED	HOW MUCH?	WHY DID I EAT IT?	TOTAL SUGAR
DAY 5				
			TOTAL	

FOOD FOR THOUGHT

In your food diary:

- Identify the 5 foods that you consumed that were highest in carbohydrates.

- Identify the 5 foods that you consumed when you were not necessarily hungry.

- Identify the 5 foods that you liked or enjoyed eating the best, even if they weren't the healthiest option.

- Identify the 5 foods that you consumed that you think were good, healthy choices.

STEP 3

The New Science
of Sugar Addiction

"The data is so overwhelming the field has to accept it. We are finding tremendous overlap between drugs in the brain and food in the brain."

—NORA VOLKOW, DIRECTOR, NATIONAL
INSTITUTE ON DRUG ABUSE

In this chapter we cover the science behind sugar addiction. It is a bit technical, as most science is, but we have summarized the key findings for you up front. If you want to know the details and are interested in learnisng more about how our brains change when we become addicted to food and other subtances, read on. If you trust us and don't really care about the details of the science, then feel free to skip to Step 4.

We are entering a new scientific era in addiction research. Up until this point, addiction has been synonymous with drugs of abuse, like cocaine and heroin. But now, more and more people are

HOW YOU FEEL	WHAT SCIENCE TELLS US
You never feel satisfied when you eat healthy food.	Your brain has been changed by constant over-eating of sugars. Dopamine, a neurochemical involved in reward and pleasure, is not functioning normally.
You feel like you need to keep eating and eating to feel satisfied.	You have developed tolerance to sugar-rich food.
You feel cranky and irritable when you are on a diet.	This is a sign of withdrawal; your brain is reacting to the lack of opioid stimulation that it is used to getting when you overeat sugars.
You constantly crave certain foods.	Your brain is reacting to the cues in your environment that are normally associated with sugar-rich foods.

developing addictions to nondrug substances and activities, which can be just as dangerous and debilitating. For example, according to psychiatrists, people can be addicted to sex, gambling, and even video games.[1] The broadening of the field isn't meant to detract from the devastation and havoc that drug addiction can cause, but rather it highlights that people's lives can be turned upside down by abuse of other things too, not just drugs.

Some people use the term *addiction* rather loosely and say that they are addicted to surfing the Web, shopping, playing basketball, or any number of things that bring them pleasure. But there is a major difference between something being pleasurable and giving us joy and something being addictive.

What Is an Addiction?

Doctors use specific criteria to assess whether a person is addicted to substances such as alcohol, cocaine, or opiates. In order to ensure that doctors follow similar guidelines when making this diagnosis, the *Diagnostic and Statistical Manual of Mental Disorders (DSM)*, a book published by the American Psychiatric Association, outlines the criteria. In order to meet the diagnostic criteria for having an addiction to drugs, one must engage in at least three of the seven criteria listed in the *DSM*, and outlined in the figure below, over the course of a twelve-month period.

As you can see from the figure, several different things happen when someone becomes addicted. A more simplistic way to view addiction can be seen in the diagram on page 61. As we review these criteria in greater depth, think about how they relate to your own behavior around food.

When a person is addicted to a drug of abuse, he ingests large quantities of the addictive substance when it initially becomes available in order to obtain the desired feelings of pleasure, or experience

SYMPTOMS OF ADDICTION

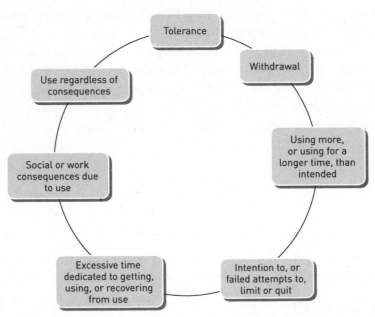

a high. This large initial consumption is sometimes referred to as a binge. The term *binge* is something that we normally think about with respect to eating, but people can binge on drugs as well. The most common binge drug is alcohol, but this can occur with illicit drugs, too.

With continued use, the brain and body develop a tolerance to the substance. This means that the person keeps taking the drug to try to experience a high, but receptors in the reward centers of the brain do not detect the substance in the same way as before, thus he needs more and more of the drug in order to feel the same high that he used to get from smaller amounts of the drug. To relate this to eating, tolerance is best demonstrated by the potato-chip phenomenon: We can't eat just one. Something compels us to want to eat more and more of them.

CYCLE OF ADDICTION

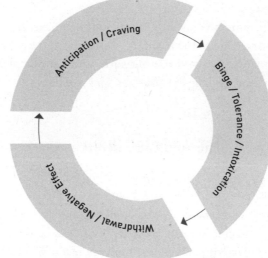

What happens if a drug addict does not have access to the drug? Withdrawal can ensue, and the addict may experience feelings of depression and anxiety, along with other possible unpleasant side effects, including nausea. Withdrawal can also be apparent in response to food. When one is dependent on excess sugars, feelings and symptoms that are similar to what one sees during drug withdrawal (such as depression, headaches, anxiety, and irritability) can arise.

In an attempt to alleviate these symptoms and satisfy his cravings for the substance, the addict may resume using the substance, despite knowing the consequences associated with this consumption. With food, cravings can be sparked by an emotional response, a habit (such as if you were accustomed to having a piece of cake after dinner most nights), or cues or reminders of a favorite food. When these events occur, our brains are reminded of how good we used to feel when eating these foods, and how that good feeling could help to ameliorate the negative feelings we face during the withdrawal phase.

All of these behaviors and conditions—bingeing, craving, withdrawal—originate in the brain. As it turns out, the areas of the brain that regulate and experience pleasure, whether that pleasure is in response to food or drugs of abuse, is very similar.

The Addicted Brain

The human brain is a complex organ with many different working parts. At any given moment, the different regions of our brains are communicating so that we can make sense of, and respond to, our environment. Different parts of our brains work together to sense stimuli, control our actions, and tell us when we need something.

Certain regions are responsible for motivation and control, feelings of pleasure and reward, and memory. These regions of the brain can sense information and communicate with each other via messengers called *neurotransmitters*. Neurotransmitters travel to, or stay away from, certain regions of the brain in response to events happening in the world around us and within our own bodies. For example, when we smell the aroma of a freshly baked apple pie, we might recall what it tastes like, decide that we want a slice, and go over and get a piece. In order for this sequence of events to occur, specific pathways in the brain need to be activated to initiate the memory of the taste of apple pie and motivate us to physically walk over to the pie and then cut ourselves a slice. Similarly, once we eat the pie, a cascade of events must occur in our brains that allow us to feel pleasure from the food, and signal to us when we have had enough and should stop eating. The figure on page 64 shows some neurotransmitters in the brain that play important roles in addiction and food intake.

When someone is addicted to a drug of abuse, these neurotransmitters are affected in key brain regions. In particular, neurotransmitters in the reward-related brain regions are influenced. *Dopamine* is a neurotransmitter that has many roles in the brain, such as being released in response to stimuli and situations that cause pleasure: having sex, eating certain foods, and consuming drugs and alcohol. We experience pleasure, in part, because of elevated dopamine levels, and thus we are motivated to continue enjoying these experiences and sensations. In other words, the pleasurable feelings that result from the release of dopamine also serve to reinforce the behavior.

Does dopamine act alone? That is, is dopamine the only neurotransmitter that plays a role in addiction? Not at all; in fact, there are a number of other chemicals in the brain that are involved in addiction. The other neurotransmitters depicted in the figure above,

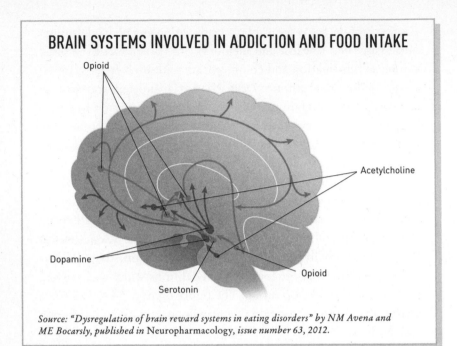

BRAIN SYSTEMS INVOLVED IN ADDICTION AND FOOD INTAKE

Opioid

Acetylcholine

Dopamine

Opioid

Serotonin

Source: "Dysregulation of brain reward systems in eating disorders" by NM Avena and ME Bocarsly, published in Neuropharmacology, *issue number 63, 2012.*

serotonin, opioids, and acetylcholine, also have roles in drug addiction and food intake or satiety (fullness), and there are numerous others that are not shown that also have contributory roles in these processes. However, our focus here is on dopamine, as it is one of the primary neurotransmitters involved in addiction, and it also plays an important role in the regulation of food intake. We need dopamine in order to motivate us to eat, to indicate whether food is safe to eat, and to tell us whether the food tastes good. If we didn't have dopamine, we wouldn't have the desire to eat (and that goes for all types of food, not just junk foods).

Now, you might be thinking that drugs and foods like sugars are clearly very different. And you're right; there is no doubt that food and drugs of abuse are very different in important ways.

However, the brain reward systems that are responsible for making drugs of abuse so addictive are actually the same pleasure systems that are activated by the foods we eat. So to our brains, the difference between drugs and some foods might not be so obvious.

The Addictive Nature of Food

One way in which foods and drugs of abuse are very different is that we need food to survive, but we don't need drugs of abuse. Interestingly, however, the survival value of food is actually one of the factors that may contribute to its addictive potential. Food is one of our basic needs, and thus our brains evolved to make us like the taste of food and seek it out when we are hungry. Some people will do some extreme things when they are faced with severe hunger (for example, theft or cannibalism), which underscores what a powerful motivator food can be. We need to eat and mate to survive as a species, so our clever brains make us enjoy those activities. That enjoyment occurs through the activation of the same reward systems that are activated by drugs of abuse. So, drugs of abuse actually hijack these primitive brain systems that reinforce natural behaviors, such as feeding. Based on this, the brain circuitry is certainly in place for foods to also become addictive, just like drugs.

Another basic factor that separates food from drugs of abuse is its availability. We have to eat food to survive, so it is all around us. Obviously, this makes drugs of abuse much different from the foods and drinks that we have available to us almost everywhere we look. In addition, there are billboards, commercials, and signs everywhere advertising food, many of which depict the types of foods that people often crave. Fortunately for drug addicts, the cues associated with drug use are less commonly seen.

Also related to availability is the fact that there are negative consequences associated with using drugs that are not seen when people abuse food. You can be arrested, fined, and jailed for buying, selling, and carrying some drugs. You can even be arrested for having an open container of alcohol in your car while driving. There is a social stigma associated with using drugs, and this is not normally the case with food (although there is a social stigma that sometimes comes with eating when an individual is overweight). So when it's proposed that certain foods with a high concentration of sugar or fast-digesting carbs in them may be addictive, what does this mean?

Well, certainly humans crave food. We need it to survive. But just because we crave these sugary, high-carb foods does not prove that we are addicted to them. Humans, especially when very thirsty, crave water, but nobody would claim that anyone has an addiction to water. If you left a person in the desert long enough and offered him water or even just showed him pictures of water, you would probably see a release of dopamine in his brain. Exhibiting this response is not sufficient to say that something is addictive. Addiction is something fundamentally different.

The New Science of Food Addiction

So far, several reasons have been discussed that suggest why food is a natural candidate to move into the addiction category. In fact, it was drug addicts (alcoholics, in particular) who first provided the hint that food intake can be an important part of the addiction cycle. In the Alcoholics Anonymous manual it says, "We now find that it is wise to eat balanced meals at regular hours. . . . The reason for this advice is simple. If we are undernourished and lack rest, we become irritable and nervous. In this condition, our tempers get out of control, our feelings are easily wounded, and we get back to the old and dangerous thought process."[2] This quote underscores what scientists have gone on to show repeatedly: disruption of the feeding cycle can contribute to addictive, drug-seeking behaviors. Since then, scientists have refined this notion and have shown that intake of certain foods, like sugars, are associated with alcohol intake.[3]

Researchers have largely looked at studies of food addiction as a way to possibly understand why there has been such a sharp rise in the rates of obesity over the last several decades. The fact that people across the globe are gaining weight rapidly cannot be explained by alterations in our genes or some sort of evolutionary change, as these changes don't happen that quickly. Instead, many suspect that the increase in obesity is due to an environmental change. Our modern-day food environment is filled with opportunities to get quick and easy access to food, which can be a good thing, but unfortunately these convenience foods tend to be highly processed, dense in calories, and high in sugars. The ease and convenience of such foods lure us to eat them or feed them to our families, but when we consume them in excess, we can experience increases in body weight.

Over the past few years, more research has investigated the idea that some foods might be addictive. The data suggest numerous overlaps between drug addiction and obesity, both in terms of behavior and brain changes. For example, studies show that when obese people are shown images of foods they desire, their dopamine system is activated as if one were showing drug paraphernalia to a drug addict. It doesn't take scientific studies to tell us this; anyone who is overweight and has gone on a diet in an attempt to lose weight can relate to the compulsion and desire to eat certain foods. That is one reason why adherence to diets is so poor: people find it almost impossible to give up the foods that they love, which are usually high in calories and contain a lot of sugars.

WHY SUGARS?

Although research has been assessing how food in general might be addictive, the foods that seem to be posing the biggest problem are not healthy food choices like leafy greens and lean meats. Rather, people with problematic eating patterns tend to consume a lot of foods made up of carbohydrates and added sugars. For the sake of brevity, we use the term *food addiction* in this book. This is meant to refer specifically to dependence–like relationships with highly palatable foods, such as those high in sugars, not just any type of food. Many people also report that they find it difficult to abstain from carbohydrates, and some feel compelled to eat them.

We see this phenomenon in the laboratory as well. Some studies suggest that laboratory animals may prefer the taste of carbohydrates to protein,[4, 5] and even prefer carbohydrates (glucose) to protein when they do not taste the sweetness that is usually attributed to its appeal.[6] Also, even when animals don't taste the sweetness of the sugar, they still show an increased dopamine response to it compared to protein.[7] Thus, it has been suggested that we may have strong and complex food preferences; even if carbohydrates don't taste great, they may still be pleasurable for us because of postingestive factors, such as signals that our gut sends to our brain, which may reinforce our consumption of them. This might explain why nonsweet carbohydrates, such as breads and pastas, are also problematic for some individuals.

DOPAMINE DOESN'T WORK ALONE

There are other reasons that support the notion that sugars could have addiction-like effects on the brain. For example, there is evidence from both human studies and laboratory studies that indicates that brain systems that regulate feeding also have a role in regulating the addiction processes. As we just mentioned, dopamine has a prominent role in addiction. However, studies show that dopamine is affected by many other things in the brain that regulate food intake. For example, in the hypothalamus (a key region of the brain related to food intake), the neurotransmitter orexin is associated with increasing food intake, but it turns out that orexin also sends information directly to the dopamine neurons in the reward systems and can promote drug seeking and addiction.[8]

There are also some satiety, or fullness, signals that circulate in the body that are associated with drug seeking. Leptin, which is a hormone that is secreted from fat cells in the body, normally works as a satiety signal by traveling to the brain to tell us to stop eating (because we have a lot of fat to store and don't need to eat more). However, when people are overweight or obese, they may become insensitive to leptin, and the receptors in the brain that normally detect these high levels of it no longer work correctly. Thus, people who have a lot of fat stored continue to eat as if they are lean. Interestingly, there are leptin receptors in the reward regions of the brain, located on dopamine neurons, and activation of these receptors can promote sensitivity to drugs of abuse.[9] A similar story is emerging for the hormone insulin, which is released from the pancreas in response to spikes in blood glucose.[10] The bottom line is that chemicals that are associated with feeding can also affect brain regions that make us want to use drugs. This adds another layer of biochemical support for the idea that certain foods may have properties of addiction.

RESEARCH STUDIES OF SUGAR ADDICTION

Most of the science suggesting that excessive intake of sugars can result in signs that resemble an addiction comes from laboratory studies conducted with rats. Although we look very different, rats are actually very good models of humans because we have similar brain systems and neural circuitry. Rats are used to study many disorders and diseases that affect humans, including those related to feeding behaviors and addictions. Pharmaceutical drugs that are developed for humans are almost always tested in rodents before they find their way into clinical trials, as rodents are generally thought to provide a good indication of what is likely to happen in humans in similar situations.

Why are rat studies important? Researchers using animal models don't have to worry about the potential influences of the environment, media, or cultures on the behaviors or brain changes they observe. It is a great way to isolate the variables of interest and minimize outside influences that could affect the results.

Several studies have been designed to assess whether aspects of addiction, such as tolerance, exist in rats offered access to sugar-rich foods or sugar solutions. Most of the time, these studies are designed to mimic the pattern of food access that might be seen in humans. Rats will have free access to water as well as a "healthy" food alternative (that is, their standard, nutritionally complete rat chow—which is sort of the equivalent to dog food, but for rats). The sugar-rich food is offered as a supplement, or treat, so that it is not the sole source of calories for the animal, and they are not forced to eat it. In some cases, this "treat" is available twenty-four hours a day, but in other cases, the rats get restricted access to it (that is, perhaps just twelve hours a day). This limited access schedule, coupled with the fact that the sugar-rich food is offered a few hours after the time that the rats typically eat (so they are hungry), leads the rats to binge on the sugar-rich food when it becomes available. After just a few weeks on this feeding schedule, the behaviors shown by the rats demonstrate some noteworthy similarities to drug addiction.[11] Rats that binge on a sugar solution consume a large amount of it when it becomes available each day, and over the course of several weeks, the amount of sugar-rich food that the rats consume increases markedly. So, already we can see that rats that overeat sugar show two symptoms that are characteristic of addiction: bingeing (evidenced by consuming a large amount of the substance in a short period of time) and tolerance (evidenced by increased consumption of the substance over time).

Another behavior apparent in rats with binge access to sugar that mirrors drug addicts is withdrawal. When deprived of sugar, rats show signs of withdrawal similar to those with opiate withdrawal; they show signs of anxiety by remaining stationary and hiding in corners of mazes, both of which are textbook examples of anxiety in rats. Other symptoms include teeth chattering, body shaking, and physiological changes, such as diarrhea and changes in body temperature. They also show signs of craving, such as ingesting more sugar when it is reintroduced following a period of deprivation. Similarly, when rats are trained to press a lever to get access to sugar, rats that previously binged on sugar that have been deprived of it will press that lever repeatedly to turn on a light above the lever that is normally on when the sugar is available, even if they don't actually get to drink any of the sugar. Thus, these rats are even willing to work for *cues* that signal sugar, highlighting how powerful food cues (such as the image that we see on a hamburger wrapper or the smell of french fries) can be when we encounter them in our environment. Collectively, these behaviors all mimic what happens in rats and people when they are addicted to drugs of abuse.

Another parallel between binge consumption of sugar and drug addiction that has been noted in rat studies is the "gateway" effect. Addiction to one drug can lead to *cross-sensitization*, meaning an increase in the likelihood that one will also become addicted to other drugs. This concept is most commonly discussed when referring to the use of drugs such as nicotine or alcohol, which some suggest may lead to an increased vulnerability to use "harder" drugs, such as cannabis, cocaine, or heroin. Well, it turns out that cross-sensitization is not reserved just for drugs of abuse; rats that overeat sugar show a cross-sensitization to other foods, particularly those high in fat, as well as drugs of abuse, such as alcohol, amphetamine, and cocaine. Thus, it appears that overeating sugars makes animals more sensitive to the effects of drugs of abuse later on. This makes theoretical sense; recall that we only have one brain reward system, and that our brain doesn't have separate systems for drugs versus foods. So, if we prime the brain system to be "addicted" to one particular substance, other addictions may ensue. As we discussed in the beginning of this chapter, there is evidence of this from research studying alcoholics, who tend to have a sweet tooth.[12]

To summarize, evidence from animal studies shows that overeating of sugars can produce a state that looks much like an addiction to drugs of abuse. Also noteworthy is the finding that animals with a history of overeating sugars more readily acquire a taste for "real" drugs later on. Changes in the brain can result from certain eating behaviors, which may then perpetuate them, creating a cycle. For example, taking certain drugs can cause people to feel a sense of pleasure or a high due to a reaction in the brain, and this positive experience may lead a person to continue to engage in that behavior, forming a cycle of addiction. Changes in brain dopamine systems have been observed in animals with a history of overeating sugars along with the addiction-like behaviors discussed earlier, and these brain changes are similar to those seen with drugs of abuse.

DOPAMINE AND EATING

Food is a natural reward and is inherently pleasurable, especially when we are hungry. Thus, it is natural for food to cause a dopamine release, but this release is normally short-lived, and it is more associated with the novelty of the food. Here is why: In addition to its role in pleasure and reward, dopamine also has an important role in learning and orienting (that is, paying attention). Have you ever consumed a food that you normally eat (for example, milk), and it tasted a little funny? Not necessarily bad, but just different? Normally, when this happens our reaction is to step back and assess the situation. Is the milk expired? Was it sitting out on the countertop for too long? A funny taste can stop us dead in our tracks and make us think about the food we are eating and reassess whether it is a good or bad idea to continue to eat it. Here is why: Our primitive ancestors had a biological drive to eat food, but getting food was not as easy as it is today (there were no supermarkets or fast-food chains), so when they acquired food, they would eat a lot of it. So, if they were to stumble upon a berry patch and they had never tasted those berries before, their dopamine systems would be activated, causing them to pay attention to what was happening in regard to this new taste, in case it were to make them sick. This way they would know to never eat it again. Rotten or poisonous food can be deadly, even in modern times, so our dopamine systems make sure that we are aware of the situation that surrounds eating new tastes, just in case.

Our brain has a lot to do to keep us moving, so in order to function efficiently, it needs to conserve energy and resources. Since we need to eat regularly, it wouldn't be very efficient for our brains to orient us in this way when eating every single morsel of food. That is why the release of dopamine is normally limited to "risky" eating, such as when a new taste is involved. Once we are used to the taste and our brains know that it is safe, the dopamine release in response to eating it decreases. This is a key neurochemical difference between food and drugs of abuse: dopamine release typically decreases following repeated exposure to a food, but it is always released when someone takes a drug.

However, studies show that when palatable foods, such as those rich in sugar, are consumed in excess, the pattern of dopamine release that is typically observed with food changes: dopamine is released in response to a sugar binge even when sugar is no longer a novel food.[13] It is as if the brain starts to treat sugar like a drug. Thus, overeating certain foods has been shown to have the potential to change the landscape of the brain, causing alterations in dopamine functioning that can affect food-intake behavior and undoubtedly contribute to the compulsion to continue to overeat.

It should be noted that there are many studies in laboratory animals that lend support to the idea that sugar-rich foods can have properties of addictions. Studies have been conducted using sugar solutions, solid foods that are high in sugar, and even foods that people tend to like to eat, such as Oreos and M&M's. In addition to the findings described above, when rats have access to these types of foods and overeat them, many engage in behaviors that are atypical, such as running over an electrified grid in order to get access to M&M's.[14] Thus, there is a growing body of evidence coming from laboratory animal studies that supports the notion that sugar-rich foods can have properties of addiction.

FOOD ADDICTION STUDIES IN HUMANS

It is important to note that not all people are addicted to sugar—many people can eat sugars and sugar-rich foods in moderation as part of a healthy diet and have no associated problems. This is similar to alcohol: if you are not an alcoholic, you can enjoy a glass of wine now and then, but you can stop drinking at any time, and you don't feel the same urge to drink that leads an alcoholic to imbibe. However, as we have seen, sugar is pervasive in modern Western diets, meaning that it takes a conscious effort and careful consideration to regulate our sugar consumption. It is relatively easy to overeat sugar-rich foods, and doing so for an extended period of time may put some people at risk for becoming dependent on them, which can lead to more and more overeating. We also have the added disadvantage that, if we become addicted to sugar, it can be tough to manage due to the constant food cues and pressures we have regarding food.

While lab-based research with rats has allowed scientists to uncover a lot of information, both behavioral and in terms of what happens in the brain, there have been several studies conducted in humans that also support the idea that overeating palatable foods can result in a state that resembles an addiction.[15] Humans eat a variety of different types of foods, many of which are rich in fats and sugars and are pleasurable to eat. In excess, however, consuming these foods may alter brain mechanisms responsible for processing rewards, potentially resulting in a hijacked brain reward system, similar to what is seen among individuals addicted to drugs, as well as the data from laboratory animal studies discussed previously.

Personal testimonies provide compelling evidence of addiction to certain foods, in particular refined or processed foods that include sugar, other carbohydrates, fat, salt, and caffeine. In fact, individuals who identify themselves as "refined-food addicts" reveal that the symptoms of addiction to these types of foods mimic the criteria doctors use to diagnose substance dependence.[16] However, while these qualitative accounts add important information to the study of the addictive nature of some foods, personal testimonies alone are not sufficient to determine the existence of an actual disorder or syndrome.

To empirically determine whether the addiction model can be applied to overeating, researchers have recently developed a survey that uses the *DSM* criteria for substance dependence; however, instead of asking individuals about drugs, the survey asks about behaviors and emotions related to food. With the use of this assessment tool (called the Yale Food Addiction Scale),[17] researchers have found increasing evidence of addiction to palatable foods in humans. Research using this newly developed scale suggests that food addiction is apparent in a variety of groups. It can be detected in individuals who are normal weight, overweight, obese, or severely obese. For instance, 41 percent of patients who are extremely obese, to the point that they are seeking surgical treatment to help them lose weight (for example, bariatric surgery), have also been found to meet the criteria for a food addiction.[18] Participants in studies that have used this scale show addiction-like symptoms such as tolerance, withdrawal, eating despite negative consequences, and failed attempts to limit consumption of certain foods. Although the scale is designed to assess addiction to food in general, not specifically to sugar, it is important to note that the foods listed as being particularly problematic to individuals are overwhelmingly carbohydrates (sugar-based foods). This supports previous research that has suggested that obese individuals with problematic eating tend to go for foods that are high in sugar.[19]

The brief questionnaire on the opposite page was adapted from the Yale Food Addiction Scale. Answer the questions and then evaluate your answers using the scoring instructions to determine whether you meet the criteria for food addiction.

What does it mean if you are addicted to food according to the scale? First, don't worry. This does not mean you are doomed to be a sugar addict forever. Once you discover the causes of your addiction and learn how to control your urges to eat sugar-rich foods, you can break free from it. The plan that we describe in part two of this book will help you wean yourself off of excess sugars and carbohydrates. We give you the tools you need to accomplish this without sacrificing eating out, socializing with friends, or other food-related events that normally derail a diet. We're going to help you handle your addiction in the chapters to come.

If you don't meet the criteria, that's fine, too. Everyone can benefit from cutting the sugar from their diet; whether you are

ARE YOU ADDICTED TO FOOD? TAKE THE TEST AND FIND OUT.

The following questions ask about your eating habits in the past year. People sometimes have difficulty controlling their intake of certain foods such as sweets, starches, salty snacks, fatty foods, sugary drinks, and others.

In the past 12 months . . .

1. I find myself consuming certain foods even though I am no longer hungry.

   0 - Never
   1 - Once per month
   2 - 2-4 times per month
   3 - 2-3 times per week
   4 - 4+ times per week

2. I worry about cutting down on certain foods.

   0 - Never
   1 - Once per month
   2 - 2-4 times per month
   3 - 2-3 times per week
   4 - 4+ times per week

3. I feel sluggish or fatigued from overeating.

   0 - Never
   1 - Once per month
   2 - 2-4 times per month
   3 - 2-3 times per week
   4 - 4+ times per week

4. I have spent time dealing with negative feelings from overeating certain foods, instead of spending time in important activities such as time with family, friends, work, or recreation.

   0 - Never
   1 - Once per month
   2 - 2-4 times per month
   3 - 2-3 times per week
   4 - 4+ times per week

5. I have had physical withdrawal symptoms such as agitation and anxiety when I cut down on certain foods. (Do not include caffeinated drinks: coffee, tea, cola, energy drinks, etc.)

   0 - Never
   1 - Once per month
   2 - 2-4 times per month
   3 - 2-3 times per week
   4 - 4+ times per week

6. My behavior with respect to food and eating causes me significant distress.

   0 - Never
   1 - Once per month
   2 - 2-4 times per month
   3 - 2-3 times per week
   4 - 4+ times per week

7. Issues related to food and eating decrease my ability to function effectively (daily routine, job/school, social or family activities, health difficulties).

   0 - Never
   1 - Once per month
   2 - 2-4 times per month
   3 - 2-3 times per week
   4 - 4+ times per week

8. I kept consuming the same types or amounts of food despite significant emotional and/or physical problems related to my eating.

   Yes / No

9. Eating the same amount of food does not reduce negative emotions or increase pleasurable feelings the way it used to.

   Yes / No

Scoring Instructions:

You meet the criteria if you answered 4 to question 1 or 2.

You meet the criteria if you answered either 3 or 4 to questions 3-7.

You meet the criteria if you answered yes to question 8 or 9.

To meet the food addiction threshold, people must meet the criteria for either question 6 or 7 and the criteria for 3 or more of the other questions (1-5, 8-9).

technically addicted or not, reducing your sugar intake is going to make a big difference to your health.

How Food Addiction Changes Your Brain

Evidence of food addiction in humans also comes from studies investigating indicators of addiction in the brain. Researchers are somewhat limited when it comes to understanding the exact neurochemical changes that occur in human brains, largely because we don't have many tools to test these changes in people. This is why the preclinical, or animal, research is so important. In order to study the brains of humans, researchers use brain-imaging techniques called functional magnetic resonance imaging (fMRI) and positron emission tomography (PET) scans. In studies that use these techniques, human participants volunteer to have their brains scanned in one of these machines (although it might sound scary, it is completely safe and painless). Functional magnetic resonance imaging technology measures blood flow in activated regions of the brain to detect neurological responses to stimuli. Positron emission tomography scans are similar but instead allow for the generation of images that show neurotransmitter receptor–specific activity occurring in the human brain.

Using fMRI technology, food addiction has been associated with increased brain activation in reward-related regions when anticipating palatable food. Interestingly, increased activation of an area of the brain called the anterior cingulate cortex was found when participants with high food addiction scores were anticipating palatable food.[20] This is similar to the type of brain activation that has been observed when cigarette smokers are shown smoking cues, like images of cigarettes.[21, 22]

Some studies have also shown changes in dopamine in reward-related brain regions in humans who are obese. Using PET technology, for example, researchers have found evidence that indicates that obese individuals may have less dopamine receptor availability,[23] a finding that has also been observed among individuals with drug addiction. This finding lends support to what is called the reward deficiency syndrome, which is based on the hypothesis that some people may have a lower-functioning reward system and, as a result, may feel as though they have to eat more to experience the reward response produced by food. A competing theory, called the hyperresponsiveness model, is that certain individuals are highly sensitive to reward, and because they may find eating more pleasurable, they engage in it more often.[24]

And it may all boil down to the genes that we are born with. Imagine that one individual is born with a dulled reward response. To be reinforced by food, he may feel that he has to consume more food than normal. This is an example of the reward deficiency syndrome hypothesis. Imagine that another individual is born with a highly sensitive reward system. Because food may be experienced as more rewarding for this individual, he may tend to overeat. This second scenario is an example of the hyperresponsiveness model. There is evidence that points toward each of these theories, which complicates the bottom line: are people overeating because their brains are overly or less responsive to reward?

To help make sense of what may appear to be inconsistent ideas, another theory has emerged called the dynamic vulnerability theory.[25] This theory proposes that an individual may be born with increased sensitivity to reward; however, after a period of overconsumption (which can be tied to both his genetics and the environment), his reward response may become dulled. This dulling of the reward response is in essence the brain change that underlies tolerance. As a result of this dulled reward response, he may continue to overeat in an effort to experience the pleasant feelings he previously felt while eating. Support for this theory comes from studies in children and adults which show that overweight individuals report increased reward sensitivity, whereas obese individuals report decreased reward sensitivity.[26, 27] Thus, it may be that initially, food is especially rewarding to some, but with increased weight and, therefore, possibly continued overconsumption, the sensitivity of their reward responses may decrease.

Another explanation for these conflicting theories may be that there is a difference between reward responses that are associated with anticipation of food and those that are associated with consumption of food, as these have been shown to vary. Evidence using fMRI technology suggests that individuals with food addiction may show more brain activation in reward-related regions when anticipating highly palatable food, but mixed responses when they actually consume the food.[28] It has been proposed that these individuals may want the food but may not necessarily like the food, perhaps due to dysfunctional reward mechanisms. For instance, some individuals may no longer experience a great feeling of reward when consuming food, perhaps due to a decrease in certain dopamine receptors, but they may still expect to be rewarded from food, so they show activation in reward regions of the brain when anticipating food nonetheless. This disconnection between wanting something but not actually liking it can also be seen in the drug abuse literature, where addicts will show great desire to obtain the drug of abuse, but the euphoria from taking it is not as great over time.[29]

It has recently been shown that sugary foods and other carbohydrates stimulate parts of the brain involved in hunger, craving, and reward. When people tasted high-glycemic-index foods, they showed greater activation in areas of the brain that regulate addictive behaviors as compared to people who consumed low-glycemic-index foods.[30] The bottom line: sugar selectively changes your brain in a way that promotes hunger and craving, and that turns on the addiction cycle.

What the Science Means

Science is now beginning to support what many people have been claiming for years: some highly palatable foods, and sugars in particular, can produce behavioral changes and alterations in the brain that resemble an addiction in some individuals. Although at first it may have seemed strange to discuss such a common and natural foodstuff in this way, the scientific evidence is mounting, and the data from research in laboratory animals and humans show that addiction to palatable foods has striking similarities to addiction to drugs and alcohol.

✳

Congratulations on making it through part one and hanging in there through all of the scientific detail. It may not seem like it right now, but understanding what's going on in your brain when you're eating sugar will help you recognize and overcome those feelings of withdrawal and craving once you start cutting it out. Get ready; part 2 is all about breaking your addiction to sugar.

FOOD FOR THOUGHT

- Identify three research findings included in this section that you find particularly interesting or that relate to your personal struggles with overeating and weight loss.

- How might understanding the new science behind food addiction make a difference in how you feel about your struggles with food?

- Were you surprised by your results when you took the food addiction quiz in this chapter? Why or why not?

PART TWO

How to Overcome Your Addiction to Sugar

STEP 4

The Sugar Freedom Plan for Breaking Your Addiction

"Sugar gives you an initial high, then you crash, then you crave more, so you consume more sugar."

—GWYNETH PALTROW

By now, you're probably beginning to understand more and more why some of your past diet attempts were doomed before they even began. Also, maybe you had never considered the possibility that sugary foods could be addictive, or maybe you weren't really ready to make a long-term change. You may now see that you're eating a lot more added sugars and other carbohydrates than you may have thought, and that you may be eating them for reasons that are seemingly out of your control. Your addiction to sugar may be derailing your weight-loss efforts, but with this insight, you are better equipped to beat it and regain control over your food choices and your body weight.

This chapter describes the Sugar Freedom Plan, which is designed to help you gradually reduce (and in some cases eliminate) the sugars and other carbohydrates that may be fueling your addiction. The plan has five phases.

PHASE	DURATION OF PHASE	WHAT IS THE FOCUS OF THE PHASE?	WHAT ARE YOU DOING IN THIS PHASE?	FOODS TO FOCUS ON
1	1–2 weeks	Sugary beverages	Cutting out completely	Soft drinks, coffee, energy drinks, fruit drinks (including 100% fruit juices), sports drinks, iced teas
2	2–3 weeks	Junk foods	Cutting out completely	Cakes, cookies, candy bars, ice cream, and foods found in vending machines
3	3–4 weeks	Carbs	Cutting out (almost) completely	Cereals, breads, pastas, rice, and other complex carbohydrates
4	1–2 weeks	Hidden sugars	Identifying, eliminating, and replacing	Salad dressings, barbecue sauces, sugary marinades, ketchup and other condiments, and sweetened peanut butter
5	Permanent change	Categories from phases 1–4	Maintaining all the changes made	Foods from phases 1–4

This plan will help you revamp your way of eating; minimize and, in some cases, eliminate the intake of foods that are addictive; and develop the strategies needed to maintain this way of eating. You have already begun some of these steps in the previous chapters by assessing your present food habits, recognizing the factors that can lead to a vicious spiral of dieting failures, and understanding the role that addiction can play in food intake.

The Sugar Freedom Plan

This approach really isn't very complicated; it's just different from diets you've tried in the past. After hearing the details of how this plan is implemented, it may remind you of other diets on the market that emphasize restricting sugar intake or carbohydrate consumption. However, there are two fundamental differences between this plan and other diets you've read about or tried in the past.

WHY IT WORKS

A main reason why this plan is fundamentally different from other diets out there is that it treats certain types of foods like drugs. By understanding the basics of addiction (which were covered in Step 3), it will be much easier for you to recognize and cope with your behaviors, feelings, and thoughts involving food, as well as react in the appropriate way to satisfy your appetite, not your addiction. You will understand what it means to be actually *hungry*, as opposed to irritable from a drop in your blood sugar. You will recognize the temporary side effects of overcoming an addiction, like withdrawal, in the initial phases when eliminating certain sugar-rich foods, and not allow this temporary discomfort to detract from your overall goals. You will recognize the cravings that you have for sugar, chocolate, and other carbohydrates in the short term as nothing more than your addiction trying to control your behavior and reel you back into a lifestyle of eating for pleasure and not for need. You will learn to use food for its original purpose—energy—and to replace the pleasure or comfort that you used to derive from food with other things in your life. You will learn how to navigate food-related situations that could be triggers for you to overeat. Just as an alcoholic learns to avoid going to bars, you will learn how to deal with the foods, food cues, and situations that may contribute to your addiction.

A second reason why the Sugar Freedom Plan works and differs from many of the other diets out there is that this is not a diet in the way that most people conceptualize diets. It's not something you do each spring for three weeks in order to squeeze back into your bathing suit; it really is a new way of eating and living. Yes, it's based on nutrition and science, but the impact on your life won't be limited to just your food intake or your weight. Once you decide to make the necessary changes in your food choices and learn how to listen to your body and feed it the foods that it *needs* (not the foods that your addiction *wants*), you will find that you can easily maintain this way of eating. And, when you see the results that it will have on your body weight and energy levels, you will be pleasantly surprised to see that not only will you be able to maintain this way of eating, but you will also enjoy it.

HOW IT WORKS

This plan is based on psychology and neurobiology. It is simple and straightforward. Step 3 explained how excess intake of certain foods can change both your brain and behaviors, much like what is seen with drug addiction. The goal of this chapter is to teach you how you can revise your approach to food and avoid common traps and pitfalls that can lead to and perpetuate addictive eating.

The core principle of the Sugar Freedom Plan is that if you restrict your intake of foods that are high in sugar and carbohydrates that quickly break down into blood sugar, you can break your addiction to sugar. By committing to changing your eating habits for the long run, you really can lose weight, and the weight loss can last. As we mentioned in Step 2, it can be time-consuming (and confusing) to determine how every food that you might want to eat will work with this plan, so we have developed the Sugar Equivalency Table (see page 195) to help decipher which foods are okay to eat, and which are not, according to the amount of sugars, fiber, and total carbohydrates they contain.

If all this talk of restricting and giving up is making you nervous, don't fret! Many people start to worry that if they have to give up all of their favorite foods, there will be nothing left to eat. Here are two promises: First, you will not starve to death if you can't have sugar-rich foods. Though it's hard to imagine, our ancient ancestors—and even those ancestors as recent as your grandmother—survived without access to Dunkin' Donuts or king-size candy bars). And second, there are *plenty* of other foods out that that are just as delicious and healthier that are just waiting to be tried.

You may be wondering, why not quit sugars and other carbo-hydrates cold turkey? Isn't that what you ultimately have to do to quit other addictions (like alcohol or smoking)? First, as mentioned earlier, although we can draw similarities between drug addiction and food addiction, they are not the same. Quitting drugs cold tur-key is not an easy thing to do. (That is why many people need to be admitted to inpatient rehabilitation centers, and even then, they are sometimes given drug-like pharmacological therapies to transition them off of drugs.) Cold turkey might work for some people, but it isn't for everyone.

Second, our food environment is such that sugar-rich foods and their cues are abundant, so trying to quit cold turkey would be extremely difficult. You would be constantly bombarded with cues and reminders of the foods that you used to overeat. Also, unlike many drug addictions, it isn't necessary to eliminate *all* sugars from your diet. Later in this book, you will see how certain sugar-containing foods, like whole fruits, can be sensible choices.

Recall from Step 1 that gradual changes are effective when trying to lose weight and establish a way of eating that can be sustainable. The Sugar Freedom Plan has been structured so that you can begin to slowly reduce the amount of excess sugars you consume, reduce your intake of other carbohydrates, and eventually come to maintain a way of eating that eliminates foods with added sugars (and empty calories) completely. The goal of this plan is to provide you with a realistic way of eating. Once you see that you can live without some of the foods that you have been overeating that you know are bad for you (for example, sodas), you will see that *you*, not your addiction, has control over what you eat. Also, you will begin to replace whatever foods you give up with healthier alternatives. We will discuss these alternatives in greater detail in Step 5, but for now, don't view the fact that you will be phasing out certain foods as though you are depriving yourself of something; instead, try to keep in mind that by reducing or eliminating unhealthy options, you are setting yourself up to make better choices.

Each of the five phases has a corresponding time frame. Note that these are meant as guides only, as some people will need more time to work through each individual stage, and some may need less. For example, in the first phase, which is geared toward eliminating your intake of sugar-sweetened beverages, if you don't really drink these already, then you probably will have no problem moving on to the next phase. But if you are one of the many people who drink sodas or other high-calorie sugary drinks (many store-bought iced teas, juices, and so on) in excess, this will likely be an adjustment for you and might require an additional week or two. However, it is advised that you stay in each phase for *at least* as long as suggested. If you rush through them, you won't be giving your brain and body enough time to adapt to the behavioral changes that you're making, and you psychologically might not have kicked the need for these foods yet. Remember, this isn't a race.

How will you know when you are ready to move to the next stage? If you get to the end of the suggested time frame and you still feel compelled to eat the foods you are restricting, stay within that phase for a little longer. You may still be experiencing withdrawal and acute cravings for these foods (we offer some strategies to overcome these two challenges in Steps 6 and 7).

Before You Start

There is some preparatory work that you should do before you start cutting out the sugar to make sure that you are ready to incorporate this new way of eating into your everyday diet. Remember that by coming this far, you have *already* taken the first steps necessary to get started. In Steps 1 and 2, you took stock of your past and present dieting habits so that you can begin to recognize where you are making mistakes and understand why your past diet attempts have failed, and in Step 3, you began to consider how some of your habits related to food intake might be promoting your addiction to food. These first steps are critical, as when you are making a life change it is crucial that you recognize *what* you are changing, and *why* you need to. If you just wake up one day and blindly decide to cut out excess sugars and other carbohydrates but don't have the background on *why* you need to do it or *what* it is doing to your brain and body, you are less likely to be able to see the value in your behavioral changes, and as a result, you will probably be less likely to stick to them in the long run.

There are a few key preparatory steps that you will need to take to make this plan work: understand sugar equivalency, learn which sugars to avoid, and assess your food stock and restock, if necessary. Let's take a closer look at each of these preparatory steps now.

UNDERSTAND SUGAR EQUIVALENCY

In order to lessen your dependence, it is not sufficient to just eliminate added sugars from your diet (although this is certainly an important step in the process). As you now know, "sugar" is not just the sugar you add to your coffee. Lots of foods that we eat are high in sugars and other carbohydrates, and even though they may not taste sweet, they can still be a problem. The first two phases of the Sugar Freedom Plan—eliminate sugary beverages and eliminate junk foods—are pretty straightforward in that most (but not all) of the foods you should avoid are pretty obvious (that is, sodas, cakes, cookies, chips, and so on). However, once you enter the next two phases—reduce carbs and, especially, reduce hidden sugars—you will need to more carefully assess the foods you eat, as it will not be so obvious whether a particular food is good or bad for you.

There are many meal-planning techniques that people implement to monitor how much sugar they eat. One popular method is to count the number of carbohydrates being consumed by looking at the grams of carbohydrates per serving. The American Diabetes Association recommends this method for people who are diabetic and trying to maintain a low-carbohydrate diet. A range of 45 to 60 grams of carbohydrates per meal is suggested (27 to 36 percent carbohydrate diet in a 2,000-calorie diet), but this can vary. Other low-carbohydrate diets require that you only eat 10 percent of your total daily calories from carbohydrates, and a low-glycemic-index diet recommends that 40 percent of your daily calories be from carbohydrates.[1] As you can see, there is a fairly large range as to what constitutes a reduced-carbohydrate diet, and it can be difficult to ascertain just how many carbohydrates you should be eating when trying to reduce them. Also, if you eat 40 percent of your daily calories from carbohydrates in the form of ice cream, is that okay? You are still sticking to the low-carbohydrates diet, right? Probably not.

Another problem is that counting carbohydrates can be tedious (you may now have a sense of this from the exercise on counting carbohydrate intake in Step 2). Keeping track of how much you consume each day and at each meal is a good idea, but, often, doing this becomes just one extra thing you need to do to stay on track with eating well, and the more you have to do to stay on track, the less likely you are to stay on track at all.

Instead of counting, it would be easier if the choice were dichotomous, or black-and-white: you simply decide to eat, or not eat, certain foods. Of course, there are disadvantages to this approach, too. First, this limits your choices. However, if sugars are causing or maintaining your addiction to food, then limiting choices is a good move; if you can't control your intake of certain foods, then maybe it is best to just stay away from them. That is part of the beauty of this approach. Once you are free of your addiction to sugars and other carbohydrates, you will end up eating less because you will be able to listen to your satiety signals and eat based on true hunger, not just pleasure. You won't *want* to overeat.

To make all of this evaluating and decision making quick and easy, John designed a new concept called sugar equivalency to help you determine which foods you should choose, or avoid, on this diet. In the Sugar Equivalency Table (see the appendix), each food is given a number based on its carbohydrate and sugar content. This simple guide tells you which foods are good choices in keeping with this diet and which are not. It should be noted that this type of analysis is not perfect. There are a variety of different factors that would have to be taken into account to develop a perfect equation, including factors that affect the rate of digestion and absorption of carbohydrates. Plus, these factors can vary depending on a person's lifestyle, behaviors, and even other foods that are consumed with the carbohydrates. Given these variables, it may be that creating a perfect formula is not even possible. But perfection or a precise calculation is probably not necessary for your purposes. Our goal here was to make this whole process less complicated, and easy to implement and use.

This table was compiled with a specific focus on identifying the sugar and carbohydrate contents of foods, but it isn't meant to replace common sense. Just because a certain food contains little to no sugar does not necessarily mean it's a healthy alternative. For example, cooking oil has a sugar equivalence of 0, but we don't recommend consuming this in excess. And when you compare chicken fat and broccoli based on their sugar equivalence (0 for the fat versus 3 for the veg), you might conclude that chicken fat is a healthier option. However, you also have to take into account factors such as the nutrients and fiber provided by the broccoli.

To calculate sugar equivalence, we took the percent of sugar that a food contains by weight (per 100 grams of food) and added 75 percent of its nonfiber, nonsugar carbohydrate weight. The idea is that starches very quickly turn to glucose (sugar) in the bloodstream, and it is this speedy sugar and carbohydrate overload that we want to avoid. Sugar equivalence is a novel, simple concept because it takes lots of data and analysis and reduces it down to one easily understood number. You can see from the table on page 94 (as well as the more expanded table that starts on page 197) that foods vary enormously in their sugar equivalency. If you are eating crackers instead of celery for a snack, for example, you are getting more than twenty times the amount of sugar equivalents for the same amount (weight) of food consumed.

Although you can modify the cutoff points based on your personal goals, as a general rule you should try to eat things under 5. Foods scoring between 5 and 10 can be consumed but in very limited quantities (and on a case-by-case basis, as some of these foods may be problematic for certain people to control). Anything over 10 should be avoided in your diet. Even if you limit your food choices to those

SAMPLE SUGAR EQUIVALENCY CALCULATIONS

FOOD ITEM (100G)	CARBS (G)	SUGAR (G)	FIBER (G)	NONFIBER STARCH (G)	= SUGAR EQUIVALENT OF STARCH	TOTAL SUGAR EQUIVALENCY
Sugar (granulated)	99.98	99.80	0.00	0.18	0.135	99.94
Honey	82.40	82.12	0.20	0.08	0.06	82.18
Raisins (seedless)	79.18	59.19	3.70	16.29	12.2175	71.41
Kellogg's corn flakes cereal	87.11	10.50	2.50	74.11	55.5825	66.08
Jams and preserves	68.86	48.50	1.10	19.26	14.445	62.95
Chocolate chip cookies (regular, higher-fat)	63.86	35.14	2.40	26.32	19.74	54.88
Archway home-style sugar-free oatmeal cookies	67.20	1.26	1.90	64.04	48.03	49.29
Popcorn (air-popped)	77.90	0.87	14.50	62.53	46.8975	47.77
Wheat bread	49.46	6.08	4.20	39.18	29.385	35.47
Ice cream cone covered w/chocolate and nuts	34.38	25.00	1.00	8.38	6.285	31.29
McDonald's vanilla triple-thick shake	26.61	20.43	0.00	6.18	4.635	25.07
Raw cashews	30.19	5.91	3.30	20.98	15.735	21.65
Plain pancakes	28.30	0.00	0.00	28.30	21.225	21.23
Cooked plain pasta	24.93	0.00	0.00	24.93	18.6975	18.70
McDonald's big mac	20.08	3.97	1.60	14.51	10.8825	14.85
Raw avocados	8.53	0.66	6.70	1.17	0.8775	1.54

with sugar equivalencies of 5 or less, you must still be mindful of your total consumption. That's because these foods still contain sugars and carbs albeit in lower amounts than many other foods. The beauty of this plan is that if you stick to eating low-sugar-equivalence foods, you won't want to overeat.

It should be noted that there are several foods with very low sugar equivalency values that are also very high in fat. This plan does not give you a green light for an all-you-can-eat, fat-rich diet. In moderation, fat can be an important part of a healthy diet, but don't lose sight of the main objective of this plan: to shift from an addictive pattern of eating to a healthy one.

AVERAGE SUGAR EQUIVALENCY OF FOOD GROUPS

FOOD GROUP	AVERAGE SUGAR EQUIVALENCY	FOOD GROUP	AVERAGE SUGAR EQUIVALENCY
Breads	33	Meat	1
Cake	44	Milk	6
Candy	66	Nuts	9
Cereals	49	Oil	0
Cheese	3	Pasta	24
Cookies	56	Potatoes	15
Dried fruit	54	Poultry	2
Eggs	1	Prepackaged dinners	13
Fast food	19	Seafood	0
Fruit	18	Vegetables	6

LEARN WHICH SUGARS TO AVOID

The Sugar Equivalency Table can be a handy tool that will help you to learn and recognize the types of foods and ingredients that you should avoid. The crux of this eating plan is to reduce and avoid sugars and other carbohydrates in your diet. However, as noted in Step 2, there are many different types of sugar out there. Which ones should you avoid, and which ones are okay to continue to consume? Which ones should be consumed in moderation?

The majority of the sugars that you probably consume come from added sugars. You will eliminate your intake of these in the first two phases of the Sugar Freedom Plan. In addition to added sugars, the other major class of sugars that you want to avoid is the kind that you consume when eating breads, pastas, cereals, and so on. These sugars will be addressed in the third phase of the Sugar Freedom Plan. Research suggests that the type of bread, pasta, or cereal that we eat can influence our blood sugar levels.[2] Whole grain bread, for example, does not increase blood glucose as rapidly as white bread. As a result, whole grain breads have a lower glycemic index than white breads. However, when looking at the Sugar Equivalency Table, you will see that most breads, pastas, and cereals, regardless of the type, are in the 20-plus equivalency range. So, if you are looking to lessen your dependence on sugar, it is best to just avoid these foods, period.

Cereals can be particularly tricky to decipher. There are some cereals that are clearly high in sugar, and unfortunately many of these are marketed toward children. Obviously, these should be avoided. In terms of the ingredients, sugary breakfast cereal drenched in milk can be remarkably similar to one of those prepackaged ice cream cones you can buy at a convenience store. Others may seem to be healthy alternatives based on the images you see on the box, but look at the labels, because they usually contain a significant amount of added sugars.

However, there are alternatives if you still really, really want to eat these types of foods. Thanks to the popularity of low-carbohydrate diets, there are many products on the market like low-carbohydrate breads and pastas. They usually have higher fiber content than traditional breads and pastas, and no added sugar. While they claim to be low-carb, and that is true in the sense that they are certainly lower in carbohydrates than other breads and pastas, they are not no-carb. So, if you do consume them, keep that in mind, and use them sparingly, if at all. It might be best to avoid them in the beginning, and as you begin to lose weight and are comfortable that you're making progress, you can try introducing a small amount of whole grain bread back into your diet and see if it makes a difference in your weight loss and feelings about food. Remember, this is not a one-size-fits-all approach. You will have to make modifications and changes, depending on your personal situation as well as over time.

Cutting back on the sugars that you know about is only half of the battle. There are also lots of foods with hidden sugars in them. As we discussed earlier, sugars come in many forms and go by many different names, so it can be a challenge to identify which foods actually contain sugars so you can avoid them and develop a strategy for making substitutes. That is why it is important to read and understand nutrition labels and lists of ingredients. Once you identify a food with hidden sugars (for example, ketchup), you can then plan for a substitution (such as sugar-free versions). We'll address these hidden sugars in the reducing hidden sugars phase of the Sugar Freedom Plan.

TAKE STOCK AND RESTOCK

The next step is to reassess your food stock. You want to be sure that you have access to the types of foods that you can eat on this plan, because you certainly don't want to be hungry for lunch and not have anything on your plan available.

If you live alone, it will be very easy to go through the kitchen and get rid of the food products that contain high amounts of sugar or that are high in simple, fast-digesting carbs; in their place, literally restock the kitchen with foods that fit with your new way of eating. However, if you don't live by yourself, you have a couple of different options. You can go ahead and throw out all of these kinds of foods in your kitchen knowing that eating only foods allowed on this diet will not only be better for you but for the health of your children, spouse, roommates, and so on. Although they will likely tell you otherwise, your kids *don't* need fruit juice to survive (they can drink whole fruit smoothies with fruit, ice, and milk), and your husband or wife doesn't need three different types of potato chips and ice cream varieties. At the least, if you are cutting out sugars, you can begin to reduce them for your family, too. Remember, you have less control over what they eat when they are away from home, so if you remove some of these options in the home, you are helping to cut back on their sugar intake. Even if your kids and spouse are not overweight, no one needs extra sugar in their diet and everyone can benefit from these items being replaced with more nutritious alternatives.

But if your spouse or children object and don't want to participate in this new way of eating, or if you live with roommates or other people who don't want to be a part of your diet revolution, then you're just going to have to use some old-fashioned self-restraint and understand which foods in your kitchen you can eat and which you can't. You might want to have a shelf in your pantry or refrigerator that is devoted to you and the foods you will eat on this plan.

Once you get rid of the foods in your kitchen that promote your addiction, identify alternative foods using the Sugar Equivalency Table and stock up on those instead. You might try some foods that are new to you. You can even take existing recipes from books and the Internet and whip them up, being sure to leave out the sugar and replace it with a healthier alternative. Many websites and online blogs now feature recipes for sugar-free and carb-free meals, and offer advice on good ingredient substitutes to make your favorite meals while adhering to your diet (we list a few of our favorite websites in the Resources section). And remember to plan ahead. Make sure you bring these healthy alternatives to work with you so that you can maintain your healthy lifestyle throughout the day. Keep vegetables and other healthy foods in the refrigerator at work instead of risking a trip to the vending machine.

Getting Started

In the following section, we outline the five phases you will use to reduce your sugar intake, each of which has a specific focus on reducing a certain category of food or drinks, an explanation of why, and a discussion of how you can do this. This section provides a bird's-eye view of what your new way of eating will look like. Because the main objective of this chapter is to outline and explain how to work through each phase, we don't talk about your alternative foods options yet, which can be key when reducing your consumption of other staples in your diet. But don't be alarmed; we have provided your substitutes in the following chapter. In fact, the rest of the book is devoted to providing you with the tools and strategies that you will need to successfully implement the Sugar Freedom Plan.

As you begin to eliminate and reduce sugar and other carbohydrates from your diet, you may experience feelings of withdrawal as well as cravings for the foods you are trying to cut out. This is normal—and it's also sometimes challenging to deal with. In Steps 6 and 7, we discuss both of these issues, explaining the science behind them and offering strategies for handling them when they come up.

Let's get started. Following are the five phases of the Sugar Freedom Plan.

PHASE 1: ELIMINATE SUGARY BEVERAGES

TIME: 1 to 2 weeks

WHY: In recent years, there has been a dramatic increase in the consumption of beverages sweetened with sugars both in the US and around the world, and some suggest that this rise in intake is associated with the obesity epidemic.[3] Additionally, the consumption of these beverages has also been shown to alter metabolism and increase the risk for type 2 diabetes, cardiovascular disease, and other conditions such as gout or dental caries.[4] There are lots of culprits out there: soft drinks, sweetened waters, coffee drinks, energy drinks, fruit drinks, and even apple juice. In fact, apple juice can be a combination of apple flavoring and 100 percent sweetener derived from concentrated fructose from the apple so it can be called 100 percent apple juice.[5]

One problem is that the size of these beverages can be very deceiving; they also can be a way in which more sugar and calories can sneak into your diet without your knowledge. A conventional 12-ounce serving of a typical sugar-sweetened carbonated beverage, for example, is approximately 150 calories. But people rarely drink one serving. In fast-food chains, convenience stores, and movie theaters, these beverages are offered in portions that can contain around 300 to 500 calories.

Moreover, while Americans have been drinking more sweetened, calorie-rich drinks, there has not been a simultaneous decrease in the consumption of other foods to compensate for the excess calorie intake. Have you ever downed a can of soda and felt full? Sugar-sweetened beverages can quench your thirst on a hot day and give you a jolt of energy from the caffeine and sugar, but they don't make you feel less hungry. It is almost as if your body doesn't account for calories when they come in liquid form. Not only do people often fail reduce their caloric intake from other sources when drinking sugar-sweetened beverages,[6,7] but drinking calories may even make you feel less full and lead you to eat more. The end result is that all of those calories obtained from drinking sodas and fruit juices are just being tacked on top of what you are eating anyway.

There is little or no nutritional value in these drinks. They seem to just add calories that turn into excess body weight. Even cutting just one serving per day has been shown to produce a weight loss of 1.1 pounds at six months, and 1.4 pounds at eighteen months.[8] That might not sound like a tremendous amount, but remember that many people are not drinking just one 12-ounce serving per day. Approximately half of Americans drink sugary beverages "on a given day," and within this half, about 25 percent derive 200 or more calories from them.[9] So, you can do the math to figure out how much weight one could lose if the average person cut out *all* of her sugar-sweetened beverages.

To put things in perspective, in 2009 Americans consumed 13.8 billion gallons of soda; the average person consumes 70,000 calories from sweet drinks each year; and research suggests that 45 gallons are consumed per person per year.[10] The bottom line is that drinking your calories may cause a host of problems that can lead to obesity and weight gain, including passive calorie overconsumption, incomplete energy compensation, and the displacement of more nutritious and filling foods.[11] This said, they seem an obvious first target for elimination. And eliminating sugary beverages is a way to reduce your caloric intake and promote weight loss without even changing your typical food-intake patterns, so it's an especially attractive first step.

HOW: If you are a big drinker of sugar-sweetened beverages, this can be a tough one. Unlike in the next four phases, going cold turkey is the best option for quitting sugar-sweetened beverages. This is because they are not a part of your new way of eating, and it is not suggested that you allow even small amounts of them into your diet. They have no value, other than giving you pleasure, which you will be getting elsewhere from now on. Make a list of all the sugary beverages you drink and create a plan for substitutes so you don't feel tempted to cheat. Pour the ones you have at home down the sink, take them off of your shopping list, and plan to buy some of the alternative drinks that we will discuss in Step 5 (see page 120).

PHASE 2: ELIMINATE JUNK FOODS

TIME: 2 to 3 weeks

WHY: Junk foods are convenient foods that we tend to grab when we're hungry and need to feel satisfaction fast; however, they often contain high amounts of fat and sugar. You'll most likely find these foods in vending machines, at sporting events, and at fast-food restaurants. However, you'll also likely find them lining the shelves of your pantry. Grocery stores have aisles of junk foods for us to purchase, and we tend to buy them as staples. We've discussed in previous chapters that these foods primarily consist of highly processed ingredients, which have little or no nutritional benefits. In fact, they are most likely fueling your addiction. It's important to identify the sources of unnecessary sugars in your diet and cut them out. As you can probably imagine, this means that you'll need to cut out sweet foods like cakes, cookies, candy bars, and ice cream as well as savory and salty foods like chips, popcorn, and pretzels, all of which are classic examples of junk food. This even includes seemingly healthy items like most granola bars, energy bars, fruit bars, caramel-laced rice cakes, and buttery crackers. The junk foods out there are seemingly endless, and they're usually sold in the middle aisles of the grocery store. You know junk food when you see it, and if you're in doubt, it's most likely junk food.

HOW: To eliminate junk foods from your diet, we recommend that you take a modified cold-turkey approach. These types of foods have no place in your diet, and you should work to get rid of them all. Much like sugar-sweetened beverages, they are very likely fueling the vicious cycle of your dependence on them. Some people can vow to eat no more junk food at this phase and be fine, but you might need to taper down your intake more slowly and eliminate these items one by one.

If you tend to eat a lot of junk food, make a list of the items that you really tend to overeat, and then use the Sugar Equivalency Table (see the appendix) to figure out which ones are highest in sugars and other carbohydrates. You can then prioritize which ones should be eliminated first. For example, if you regularly eat high-sugar-equivalency items such as coffee cake and candy bars and have a pair of prepackaged cupcakes for dessert every night, phase these out first. Once you're confident that you've moved past them, target other items on your list and cut them out next. Work your way down your list of common junk foods until you have eliminated them all. We allowed two to three weeks for this phase, but you might need less or more time depending on how much of these foods you eat.

The key to cutting out junk foods is replacing them with healthy alternatives (not substituting them with other junk foods). In the next chapter, we'll help you identify some substitutions for these and the other types of foods that are being reduced so you'll be prepared and less apt to regress to old eating habits. However, it may take some experimenting on your part to figure out which types of foods work for you to keep you full without compromising on taste. Also, we will discuss how to manage and mitigate withdrawal symptoms that may emerge when you begin to cut out a large portion of your sugar intake.

PHASE 3: DRASTICALLY REDUCE CARBS

TIME: 3 to 4 weeks

WHY: When you reach this point, pat yourself on the back and congratulate yourself! You have eliminated the sugar-rich, empty calories from your diet. At this point, you should start to see and feel a change: you have fewer withdrawal symptoms and more energy, and there is a noticeable difference in the way that you look and feel about yourself. Not only have your disrupted the cycle of dependence, but you have also proven to yourself that you can be in control of what you eat. However, the work does not end here. While you have reached a milestone, it is important to continue on and lessen your dependence on other types of carbohydrates that are often overconsumed.

Simple and complex carbohydrates were described in Step 2. While you have already reduced your intake of simple carbohydrates, like sugars from beverages, you still have to tackle complex carbohydrates, like breads, pastas, and rice. Recall that both simple and complex carbohydrates affect your blood sugar in ways that can detract from your weight loss. If you eat them in excess, you will soon be craving other foods, often those that are high in sugar or largely consist of other carbohydrates. Eating too many carbohydrates is like putting yourself on a roller coaster; your blood sugar zooms up shortly after you eat, then goes crashing down after a short time. Before you know it, you're hungry because your body quickly digested the food; you're craving more, and so the ups and downs continue. There is a way to get off of the roller-coaster ride and take control: reduce your intake of any carbohydrates that you abuse, and by *abuse*, we mean eating them not necessarily because you need them due to hunger, but because you want them to feel normal and to avoid the awful feelings associated with the withdrawal syndrome.

HOW: The process of cutting back on bread, pasta, rice, and so on will probably take more time than the previous two stages. This is largely because many people are heavily dependent on these types of complex carbohydrates as the primary constituents in many meals. Instead of having toast for breakfast or a sandwich for lunch, you will need to come up with alternatives. Instead, you may opt for eggs and fruit for breakfast, and a large green salad with chicken on top (hold the croutons and the sugar-laced dressings) for lunch. Thinking of whipping up some mac and cheese for the family for dinner when you get home from work? Think again—you will need to find a healthy, low-carbohydrate alternative. Maybe you can broil a nice piece of fish and serve it with a side of microwave-steamed vegetables (the preparation time for the mac and cheese and the fish and vegetable dinner are probably comparable).

As with junk foods, a good strategy is to list the carbohydrates that you tend to overeat most, and then cut them out one by one. Make it a rule of thumb that once you cut something out, you cut it out for good. If you follow that strategy, you'll gradually chip away at that list of foods that you want to eat less of. We recommend that you phase out breads and pastas first, then move on to cereals (unless you are eating lots of highly sweetened cereals, in which case you should cut those out first, as they are loaded with added sugars). Next, phase out rices and other starches. Take it one step at a time. Remember, this is a process, and you are phasing these foods out of your life while, at the same time, replacing them with others. For example, instead of having two cups of spaghetti for dinner, try having one cup and topping it with some lean meat to complete your meal. Eventually, you could replace the pasta with a vegetable—squash is a great substitute. Or have a hot dog but without the bun (and add an extra helping of vegetables on the side or as an appetizer). By making small changes as you feel ready and continuing to keep track of what you're eating, you'll find yourself transitioning to a new way of eating with ease.

PHASE 4: REDUCE HIDDEN SUGARS

TIME: 1 to 2 weeks

WHY: Dressings, sauces, and condiments may seem to merely add some flavor to your food, but they often add sugars that can work against your weight-loss goals. A small amount of some condiments can add whole grams of sugar to your meal. Furthermore, we usually don't use only one packet of sweet-and-sour sauce or ketchup; instead, we douse our food in these sugar-rich add-ons. Consequently, you might think that you're doing all you can to reduce the amount of sugars you're consuming, but that might not be the case if you continue to eat foods with hidden sugars.

Note that there are many foods that appear to be "diet" foods that actually might be bad to eat for your new eating plan. Many foods labeled as "diet," "low-fat," or "no-fat" replace the fat content with more carbohydrates. We tend to see "low-fat" and think this is a healthy option, but if "low-fat" is a synonym for "high-sugar," then it is clearly a no-no.

There are also products on the market now that are labeled "sugar-free," which appeal to people who are either diabetic or trying to restrict their sugar intake. Proceed cautiously with these products as well. While these products may indeed be sugar-free, they may still contain a lot of fast-metabolizing carbohydrates. Sugar-free cookies are the best example of this. You might think that according to this diet plan, you could eat an entire box of sugar-free cookies and feel guilt-free. Nothing could be further from the truth. The good news is that if you did eat a box of sugar-free cookies, you would have avoided consuming the 100 to 200 grams of sugar that might be in a box of regular cookies. The bad news is that you may have consumed as much as 400 or 500 grams of carbohydrates. In other words, you didn't consume any sugar, but you might as well have! While implementing this plan and researching the foods that you like to eat, you'll be shocked to find that many foods and condiments that you never suspected, including ketchup and barbecue sauce, contain sugar.

HOW: You may find, as you progress from one phase to the next, that reducing hidden or lesser-known sugars goes more smoothly than previous phases. This is because you'll already have established healthy eating habits and be used to making substitutions for the foods that you used to overeat. The goal here is to use your knowledge of nutrition labels to identify the foods that you eat which contain hidden sugars and to identify sensible replacements for them, like the ones we suggest in the next chapter.

PHASE 5: MAINTAIN YOUR NEW WAY OF EATING

TIME: The rest of your life

WHY: As we mentioned in the introduction, the Sugar Freedom Plan is a *way* of eating, not a temporary diet. That means once you cut out these sugary, carb-rich foods, you'll continue eating this way for the rest of your life. If you only eat this way temporarily and eventually go back to your old ways of eating, you can be certain that the addiction will rope you back in pretty quickly. The four phases just described lay the foundation for a healthy eating style that you can maintain forever. The key to achieving your goals lies in your knowledge of where sugars exist and what you can replace them with, and the consistent desire and dedication to follow what you know.

HOW: As we mentioned at the beginning of this section, each phase takes time. Follow the allotted time guidelines—as a *minimum*. Be patient with yourself. If you find that one phase takes longer than what is listed or than you expected, that's fine! The important point is to achieve the goal of that phase, not how quickly you do it. Try to identify why certain phases are more difficult than others. This may help you to troubleshoot and figure out ways to transition through that phase that are specific to your needs. Invest the time you need; it will be well worth it in the long run.

Elimination versus Reduction

This eating plan can only be as strict as you make it. There are dozens and dozens of absolutely delicious foods that are acceptable to eat on this diet, so in that regard, the diet really isn't restrictive at all. However, this diet is strict in that it advises that most sugars and other carbohydrates be removed from or drastically reduced in your diet. While we provide the tools that you need to recognize where sugars are and how to avoid them or use alternatives, as well as how to overcome your addiction to them, it can still be difficult to avoid eating sugars. This is largely because in the world of processed foods and fast-food restaurants, added sugars and carbohydrates lurk in almost every prepared food.

So, you'll have to keep in mind that the modern food environment isn't necessarily friendly toward your new way of eating. Forget easily finding a food or beverage that fits this diet in a convenience store or vending machine. Even if you shop in a modern, large grocery store, processed foods have so overtaken the aisles that it may take some maneuvering to fill your cart with only the foods that fit into this way of eating. For example, grocery stores or supermarkets have entire aisles dedicated to cookies, cakes, and crackers, which are forbidden on this diet. They have an aisle for breads and pastas, which are also on the no-no list. Then there's the aisle for beer, which probably is not a good idea as it is nothing more than a liquid carbohydrate. The frozen food section has TV dinners, which, when you read the nutrition labels, you'll find are heavily dosed with carbohydrates and sugar. And don't even think about going into the bakery section. The point is that you will need to plan out your shopping trips to avoid the aisles that contain the foods that you're trying to avoid. The two areas of the grocery store where you'll spend most of your time shopping are the produce section for fresh fruits and vegetables and the meats and seafood section.

So, let's say you have gone through the Sugar Freedom Plan, are happy and healthy, and have reached your weight goal. Life couldn't be better. You feel in total control of your food choices. You no longer eat foods for emotional reasons or rely on them in part to make you happy. You are the boss. So, can you now have a piece of cake at your kid's birthday party or at a holiday work event?

The answer to this question really depends. On the one hand, you now have alternatives that take the place of sugar- and carbohydrate-rich foods, so why risk relapsing and falling back into your old ways of overeating? Again, this book is not designed to introduce yet another diet plan; it is designed to offer suggestions for sustainable lifestyle changes. Therefore, although you may have completed the Sugar Freedom Plan and feel great about your body and in your body, that does not mean you should ditch all of your efforts just to return to this book or another diet book in a year.

With that said, making all foods that contain sugars and fast-digesting carbohydrates off-limits is easier said than done, especially in today's food environment. As mentioned earlier, it's not just the obvious culprits like soda and candy that contain these ingredients but also foods that seem like healthy options (certain iced teas, energy bars, and so on). Our intention is not to ban all sugar from your diet—if that were the case, we all would probably have to start farms in our backyards and learn to live off the land. Plus, some foods like fresh fruits contain natural sugar but are a healthy choice. Instead, this book advocates a diet free of the major sources of added sugars, like many desserts, sodas, and snack items, and calls for a drastically reduced overall intake of carbohydrates.

So, the answer to this question is not necessarily very clear-cut; it depends on factors specific to your circumstances. You know yourself. You know if you can eat a piece of cake at a birthday party and continue to implement a low-sugar diet or if this decision will completely derail you. If you're concerned that you may not be able to introduce a high-sugar food back into your diet without comprising your goals, then don't. You may feel more confident a week, a month, or a year from now, but don't risk it if you don't feel fairly confident that you can maintain your healthy way of eating afterward.

No Bland and Boring Diet Food Here

People who have tried restricting their sugar intake on other low-carbohydrate diets have complained in the past that initially the foods they were allowed to eat seemed boring. It's hard to imagine someone saying this when you consider all of the vegetables there are, how many fruits fit into the diet plan, and how many meats and seafood options are available—and how many different ways these foods can be prepared. You don't need to be a professional chef; given this variety of ingredients, anybody with a morsel of talent around a kitchen can come up with an unlimited number of recipes using different spices and sauces that can result in tastes and flavors too enumerable to list. Given these possibilities, your food really doesn't have to be boring—even if you're a vegetarian (see box on page 135).

The people who complain about the options being boring when on a low-carbohydrate diet may really be saying something completely different. Well, *they* may not be saying it: this may actually be their *addiction* talking. Have you ever seen someone who has recently quit drinking alcohol drinking an O'Doul's alcohol-free beer at a party? They often complain that the O'Doul's tastes boring. Or have you seen someone who's trying to quit smoking take puffs from one of these electronic vapor cigarettes? Again, often these people describe the experience as boring. It is likely that what they're describing as boring is the fact that neither the O'Doul's beer nor the electronic cigarette fully satisfies their addictive craving for alcohol or nicotine. When you drink real alcohol, you get a buzz, and when you smoke real cigarettes, you ingest a lot of nicotine. Both alter reward-related neurochemicals in your brain, making you feel good and leaving you feeling anything but bored.

The same thing happens with food. So, when you restrict your consumption of addictive substances and replace them with something else, the experience may feel boring compared to what you are used to experiencing. If you crave certain foods, you may find it difficult to get them out of your mind. When addicted, you can develop tunnel vision toward the object of desire, and entertaining the thought of other foods might be difficult.

So, if this diet initially seems boring to you, it probably is your addiction speaking. Give it time. As your addictive cravings subside and you regain control over your eating habits, not only will you will be less focused on those foods that you know are bad for you, but eventually you will also rediscover the wonderful flavors of other types of food.

No Calorie Counting Required

You might be wondering: Do I have to count calories? The good news is no. This plan isn't structured around counting calories. This makes it easy to adhere to and gives you one less thing to worry about in your life. The reason why you don't have to count calories is because you can eat as much as you like. This is a bold statement, and not one that you will often read in many diet plans. How can this be the case? The reason is really quite simple. If you stick to foods that are free of sugar and carbohydrates, you will find that you no longer *want* to overeat.

Our natural satiety signals generally work really, really well when they aren't being squashed by the powerful urges that may result from an addiction to food. When you are addicted to sugar, you bypass or ignore these satiety signals, which leads you to eat more than you need and you gain weight. Your body only *wants* you to eat as much as it needs to function, but if you're addicted to food, your addiction may lead you to eat more than you need. When you reduce your intake of the foods that promote your overeating, you'll inevitably decrease your caloric intake and lose weight. Further, the quality of the calories you will likely consume will be better than before, and this will also assist you with your weight-loss goals.

How Exercise Fits In

We have so much going on in our lives that exercise (along with eating right) often ends up on the back burner. Instead of seeing exercise as something that brings us pleasure, it becomes something that we never seem to have time to do and we end up feeling guilty about it. Exercise should be something that you *want* to do, not necessarily something that you *have* to do.

Also, your overeating of sugars and other carbohydrates may result in periods of withdrawal, which may leave you feeling lethargic, anxious, annoyed, and tired. The dips in blood glucose levels that you experience from bouts of excess sugar intake will add to these feelings of lethargy. Once you reduce the amount of sugars that you consume and lessen your dependence on them, and as a result get rid of the side effects of lethargy, you may actually look forward to exercising. You don't have to be a cycling fanatic or wear a sweatband to Zumba class, exercising can be as simple as taking a walk in your neighborhood, biking with a friend, or going for a swim.

There are several reasons, aside from weight loss, that exercise is important. If exercising with weight loss as your goal has not been effective in the past, you may find some new motivation in recent scientific studies. Your mind can benefit tremendously from regular exercise. For example, studies using animal models have shown that exercise can result in the development of new neurons in the brain and can also improve memory.[12] Studies in humans provide evidence that exercise may affect mood. For instance, evidence suggests that exercise may help to reduce depression, stress, and anxiety,[13] which, one might argue, may also help to reduce emotional overeating.

In the beginning phases of this diet, you may experience symptoms of withdrawal, which we will cover in more depth in Step 6. During this time, there is nothing like exercise to make you feel better. While exercise may not seem appealing to you at the time, you will definitely feel better if, as Nike says, you "just do it!" Also, there is a biological basis for exercise being rewarding. Have you ever heard of a runner's high? When people exercise, chemicals called endorphins are released in their brains, and these chemicals are associated with pleasure. But exercise doesn't always feel good when you first start a regimen. Studies measuring endorphin levels during exercise found that they were the highest when participants finished exercising,[14, 15] indicating that endorphin release increases with activity, which may explain why the first few minutes of exercise can seem the hardest to get through. Once you start moving and the endorphins start flowing, you feel good.

Here is another reason why exercise is important: Once you kick your addiction to sugar, you may find that you feel the urge to replace the pleasure that you used to derive from food with something else. This is actually a well-known concept in the addiction literature, referred to as addiction transfer. Most commonly, this concept is discussed within the context of drug addiction, wherein an addict might transfer from one drug addiction to another. Have you ever been to an Alcoholic Anonymous meeting? People at these meetings are sometimes heavy smokers and coffee drinkers. This is a perfect example of addiction transfer. They replace their addiction to alcohol with other (not ideal) addictions to nicotine and caffeine.

The same thing may happen with addiction to food. There is some evidence that when people quit compulsively overeating, they turn to other unhealthy substitutions. For example, a trend has been observed in which people who experience dramatic weight loss following bariatric (gastric bypass) surgery are at risk for substance abuse.[16, 17]

It's obviously not healthy to substitute one addiction for another, but it is advisable to replace an unhealthy source of pleasure with a healthier one, such as exercise. Remember, palatable foods and exercise can both activate reward systems in the brain, so perhaps you can replace the pleasure that you used to get from eating excess sugars and other carbohydrates with the pleasures of exercise. Sound too good to be true? It isn't. You may find that you will welcome exercise because once you've lost weight and you've gotten your food intake under control, you'll feel better and you'll have more energy.

Simple thermodynamics says that if you're more active and burning more calories while maintaining the same amount of calorie consumption, you will lose weight. But again, forced exercise is not the key. The worst way to get someone to exercise and participate in sports is to tell them that they *have* to do it. But we certainly encourage you to incorporate walks, bike rides, or whatever other activities you find fun into your routine, even for just thirty minutes each day to get you moving. Try not to view it as a chore, but rather as way to make your weight-loss goals happen even faster. Not only will you burn calories, but you will also tone your muscles and feel better about yourself.

*

By now, you probably have a good idea of which foods you should avoid, but you may still have a lot of questions as to which foods you should eat instead. These details and specific examples will be discussed more fully in the next chapter, but in brief, as you progress through the Sugar Freedom Plan, you will move away from a diet dominated by sodas, junk foods, breads, and pastas, and instead move to a diet in which you'll eat things like chicken, beef, fish, seafood, pork, nuts, whole fruits, vegetables, and eggs. Most of these foods are very high in protein and contain almost no sugar or other carbohydrates. Because of their high protein content, these types of foods are more satiating, which means that, when you eat them, you'll stay full—and feel full—for a longer period of time than you would if you were eating carbohydrates. How does this happen?

Well, when we eat, satiety signals are released from our stomach and intestines that tell our brains we have had enough. There is evidence to suggest that our satiety signals function less effectively following the overconsumption of sugars,[18] and a number of studies have reported that protein intake results in increased satiety compared to consumption of carbohydrates.[19] The beauty of this plan is that you will not want to overeat these foods in the way that you might overeat carbohydrates, because they are satisfying, making you feel full, and you aren't eating these foods for the hedonic pleasure that might drive the overconsumption of sugars.

It is true that fatty foods, including certain meats, are more calorically dense, which means they typically have more calories per serving than some foods high in carbohydrates. But, from this, you cannot conclude that eating fatty foods will make you fat. This was the erroneous conclusion of many who adopted the fat-free weight-loss plan. As a result of cutting out fat, many people ended up eating more carbohydrates, much more than one should eat if one wants to lose weight. Also, when you eat low-carbohydrate, high-fat foods, your glucose and insulin levels don't spike and quickly decrease as they can with some carbohydrates, so it is less likely that you will be hungry soon after eating.

However, just because you don't have to count calories doesn't mean you should abuse that privilege. You still need to be mindful of what you are eating. You should think about an appropriate portion size for the foods you're eating and reflect on how satisfied you feel after eating them.

One of the big benefits of the Sugar Freedom Plan is that over the course of approximately two to three months (for most people), you will wean yourself from your dependence on added sugars and excessive carbohydrates. As this happens, you'll begin to see and feel changes in the way that you approach food. No longer will you want to binge eat, stuff your face, or think that you have to eat gut-busting amounts of food in order to feel satisfied after every meal. You'll begin to let your satiety signals do their job and tell you when you have had enough. Your food intake will be dictated by your stomach, not an unhealthy relationship with food. So, as you overcome your sugar addiction, you can expect to eat smaller portions of food and thus weight loss can ensue. In addition, as you lose weight, you'll find that you concurrently lose your cravings for sugars, and your desired portion sizes will decrease. Remember, on average, the less you weigh, the fewer calories you need to maintain your weight, so your body will ask you for less food as time goes on and as you continue to lose weight.

You will see that once you lose your cravings for food, which are caused by your addiction, your life will no longer revolve solely around eating and obsessing about food. You'll finally believe that it is possible to settle down to three square meals a day, with a couple of small snacks in between—a meal pattern that in the past may have seemed like an impossibly small amount of food to eat. You'll eat enough so that you can go about your daily routine, but your daily routine will no longer involve obsessing about food.

Are you wondering how you're going to do all of this? In the next chapter, we will discuss how to begin this process and offer specific suggestions of foods and drinks that are encouraged within this eating plan.

FOOD FOR THOUGHT

After reading through each of the five phases outlined in this chapter, which phase(s) do you think may be the most difficult for you, and why?

Think of at least one strategy that may be helpful for you as you seek to accomplish each goal.

- What strategy can you use to eliminate sugary beverages?
- What strategy can you use to eliminate junk foods?
- What strategy can you use to reduce carbohydrates?
- What strategy can you use to reduce hidden sugars?
- What strategy can you use to maintain your new way of eating?

STEP 5

What to Eat and What *Not* to Eat

"Thou shouldst eat to live, not live to eat."

—SOCRATES

U p to this point, most of what has been discussed has been somewhat bad news: diets usually fail, sugary foods can have properties of addiction, and you have to quit eating certain foods that you think you love. Unfortunately, sometimes the truth is a bitter pill to swallow. If you're depressed from hearing about the doom and gloom, then this is the chapter that you've been waiting for.

This is the chapter where you learn about the kinds of foods that you *can* eat. Once you know *what* to eat, an equally important question is what you should do about the foods you still desire but know you should now avoid. Avoiding foods can be difficult, especially in our modern food environment where sugar-rich, high-calorie foods have become a staple. This is where substitutions and alternative foods come into play; they are key to your new way of eating. This chapter will review some of the primary foods that you should stay away from in order to reduce your dependence on sugars and suggest appropriate alternatives that you can eat to satisfy your cravings. You'll see that eating the right foods can actually be pretty easy, especially once you discover some appropriate alternatives to those foods that feed into your addictive overeating.

Note that if you are truly addicted to sugars (you can tell by taking the self-assessment on page 77), you will most likely have to work a little bit harder to stick to this way of eating than someone who doesn't have a strong addiction. This is because you aren't just battling the urges that one might normally experience when limiting certain foods on a diet; you are also fighting the cravings and experiencing the withdrawal that may come along with your addiction, which is driven by biological impulses and can impede your progress. But don't worry; in Steps 6 and 7, we'll cover how to recognize and deal with aspects of withdrawal and craving.

Think about the following suggestions about the types of food to eat as a general guide. Your personal nutrition needs and food preferences should also be taken into account whenever making food choices so that you can tailor the foods that you eat accordingly. The goal of this book is to inform you about the aspects of addiction that can manifest in response to overeating some types of highly palatable foods so that you can use this information to reconsider your eating habits and enact the necessary changes in what you eat to ensure that you are in control of what you eat. This chapter offers some suggestions, not a prescription, of healthy alternatives to foods that you may crave. It will ultimately be up to you to figure out the best eating plan that will work specifically for *you*. But here are some ideas to jump-start the process!

Let Go of Liquid Sugars

In Eliminate Sugary Beverages, you'll bid adieu to liquid sugars (beverages sweetened with sugars). As you now know, many of our excess calories come from beverages. In fact, studies show that not only is the consumption of calorie-dense beverages on the rise, but also that when you drink your calories, your body elicits a very different response than when you eat solid foods. The bottom line: liquid calories appear less satiating.[1]

By avoiding sugar-sweetened beverages, such as colas and other soft drinks, and replacing them with some of the alternatives described below, you can drastically reduce the amount of sugar you take in. Note that many drinks that look healthy, like sports drinks or iced teas, contain a lot of sugar, and so it's important to remember to check the nutrition label before drinking.

It's important to drink a lot of liquids, and water is without a doubt the best thing to drink for your health. In fact, it's a good idea to get in the habit of carrying a bottle of water with you throughout the day. Tea and coffee may be acceptable options as well, as they have sugar equivalencies close to 0, but this assumes that you sweeten them with artificial sweeteners (which we will discuss in the next section). If you enjoy your tea or coffee with cream or milk in it, watch out! Both cream and milk contain sugars.

If you insist on drinking sodas, think about what it is about the soda that you like. Some people are attracted to the carbonation or fizz. If that is you, opt for seltzer water. It is carbonated, but calorie- and sugar-free, and can come in lots of different flavors. Mineral water is also a good choice; it comes in fizzy and still versions. You may want to use diet sodas and beverages sweetened with artificial sweeteners (including teas and coffees) with caution, in light of the information we discuss next. It turns out that they don't necessarily reduce obesity and may not help to reduce your dependence on sugars.

What about Milk?

Milk is usually a household staple. Whether you start the day with a big bowl of cereal and milk, use it to cool off your first cup of coffee, down a large glass with your bacon and eggs, or cap off dinner with dessert and a cold glass of milk, like most Americans you probably have a gallon of milk in your refrigerator.

And guess what? Milk has sugar in it! Plain cow's milk purchased in your local grocery store doesn't contain added sugar; *lactose* is the type of sugar that occurs naturally in milk and other dairy products, such as cheese. Switching to skim doesn't help matters much. Skim cow's milk has reduced fat content, which reduces the calories, but the lactose amount is the same. If you purchase flavored milks, such as chocolate or strawberry, sugar is added to increase sweetness. Alternative milks such as almond, soy, or oat milk may also contain added sugar, so be sure to check the nutrition label.

Cow's milk has a sugar equivalency of 5 (see the Sugar Equivalency Table in the appendix). It's not a very high number, and that's because it's mostly comprised of water. Also, there are nutritional advantages to dairy products that may contain lactose that are important, such as calcium and vitamin D that help to promote bone health, which makes drinking milk and consuming other dairy products acceptable. Now, there are lactose-free options available, including lactose-free milk and other dairy products and light versions of soymilk, that contain, or are fortified with, vitamins and minerals such as calcium and vitamin D. Again, be sure to read over the nutrition label to check for the amounts of sugars and carbohydrates contained in these products.

Bottom line: If you must drink milk, limit the amounts of it, and measure how much you use. If you are one of those people who sips coffee throughout the day, be aware that when you pour your milk directly from the jug, gauging the amount you drink can be tricky. Most creamers should be avoided, as they contain a lot of sugar, but there are some sugar-free creamers available.

Fruit Juices

Avoid fruit juices as beverages, as one big glass of fruit juice can contain as much sugar as ten or twelve pieces of the fruit. Also, some fruit juices have added sugars, like high-fructose corn syrup or sucrose, to make them even sweeter. In addition, fruit juices don't have the fiber and some of the nutrients that you get in whole fruits. Dried fruits are also something to be careful about consuming, as many have added sugar.

Sugar Substitutes

The big question on your mind may be this: if I am going to remove sugars from my diet, can I substitute alternative or artificial sweeteners to sweeten my beverages and meals? As you now know, sugar isn't just the white stuff you put in your coffee; common table sugar substitutes, like honey and molasses, are also considered sugars, and it doesn't help much to substitute one sugar with another.

This is really a difficult question to answer. On one hand, the goal is to reduce your intake of sugars and your dependence on them, so instead of using substitutes, you should perhaps focus on alternative foods. We know that the taste of sugars, and even the effect that they have once they hit our stomachs, can independently activate the brain reward systems. So, when you consume a sweet substitute, like aspartame, you could still be satisfying your addiction. However, this doesn't necessarily mean that sugar substitutes are always a bad idea. Just like morphine addicts sometimes need to take methadone to help them get clean, perhaps artificial sweeteners can help in the beginning stages of weaning you off of high-sugar, high-calorie foods.

There are many artificial sweeteners available that are used to sweeten a variety of drinks and foods without the added sugars or calories. But the question is, do they cause addiction like carbohydrates and added sugars can? The answer is probably not. Artificial sweeteners are, by definition, artificial. This means that while they can activate some of the hormones and neurochemicals in our body that are associated with ingesting real sugars, they don't do it to the same extent. If you recall, one study reported that mice preferred glucose to protein even when they could not taste it, suggesting that factors aside from taste (for example, postingestive effects) may be involved in the rewarding effects of sugar. Similarly, when rats were trained with and given access to both glucose and an artificial alternative (saccharin) but the taste of the glucose was modified by adding an unpleasant taste to it, the rats still preferred glucose.[2] It appears that real sugars may have a stronger effect on our reward systems, and thus, may be more likely to contribute to addiction.

There has been a lot of buzz about the safety of artificial sweeteners (also referred to as nonnutritive sweeteners, because they have few, or no, calories), such as aspartame, saccharin, neotame, and sucralose. Besides being found on restaurant tabletops, ready to be added to a cup of coffee, they are often contained in some soft drinks, ice creams, cookies, jellies, yogurts, nutrition bars, and many other foods. Considering that these artificial sweeteners are becoming increasingly commonplace in our diets, one is left to wonder: are they safe?

Among the media, there is widespread concern about the effects of artificial sweeteners on health, and with good reason. There are a handful of studies that suggest that artificial sweeteners might not be as safe as one might think; studies have linked aspartame and saccharin to cancer,[3, 4] and identified sucralose as a migraine trigger.[5] However, there are several other studies suggesting the opposite, finding that they are safe. The FDA states that artificial sweeteners do *not* cause adverse reactions. Similarly, with regard to aspartame, the American Cancer Society reports "no health problems have been consistently linked to aspartame use." However, both do call attention to the fact that people with phenylketonuria (PKU), a rare genetic disorder in which people are unable to break down the amino acid phenylalanine, should limit their intake of phenylalanine from all sources, including aspartame.[6] Based on this evidence, artificial sweeteners are considered safe.

You might also wonder whether or not there are potential health benefits from consuming artificial sweeteners. With regard to weight loss, there is very limited evidence to suggest that the use of artificial sweeteners leads to decreased calorie consumption or weight loss. In fact, some research suggests that consuming artificial sweeteners is linked to, and might promote, obesity![7] The American Heart Association and American Diabetes Association state that the data are inconclusive as to whether replacing caloric sweeteners (such as sucrose) with artificial sweeteners is beneficial for energy balance or cardiometabolic risk factors.[8] In other words, it is *not* clear if consuming artificial sweeteners helps with weight loss, energy balance, or risk factors having to do with our hearts and metabolism.

So, before you sprinkle NutraSweet and Equal into your coffee and think it helps you to lose weight, think again. But if you are having a tough time reducing your intake of sweets, artificial sweeteners may be able to help you transition from eating high-sugar, calorie-laden foods and get accustomed to this diet plan. However, remember that artificial sweeteners can affect brain reward systems in ways that are similar to sugars. So, if you find that they hinder your progress by triggering cravings for more food, then it might be better to avoid them completely.

What to Eat Instead of Junk Food and Other Carbs

For many of us, our diets are dominated by carbohydrates. When you give up junk foods, breads, and pastas, what else can you eat? In this section, we will go over some alternatives that are not only healthy but will also leave you feeling satisfied.

VEGETABLES

Vegetables should, without a doubt, be your new go-to food. Vegetables should make up a big portion of what you eat. You want to try to fill up on these nutritious, low-calorie foods. The general rule is the greener and the leafier the vegetable, the lower its sugar equivalency and the better it is for you to eat. Vegetables are great because most of them have low sugar equivalencies and can be great snacks or complement a meal when served as side dishes. Broccoli, cauliflower, or zucchini, which you can top with butter or Parmesan cheese, all work great.

Are there any vegetables that should be avoided? While for the most part vegetables are a great thing to eat when trying to control your intake of sugars and other carbohydrates, some vegetables are starchy and should be used in moderation, or just not consumed at all. For example, winter squash (including acorn and butternut) are high in carbohydrates. In fact, 1 cup of acorn or butternut squash provides, on average, approximately 15 grams of carbohydrates. Similarly, corn is high in carbohydrates relative to other vegetables, as are many legumes, like black-eyed peas, green peas, or split green or yellow peas. Starchy beans, including all varieties of lentils and black, white, kidney, pinto, garbanzo, and refried beans, are another group of high-carbohydrate vegetables.

However, as with fruits (discussed next) and dairy, although these foods do contain sugars, the amount is certainly less than what you would find in junk food. Further, they are usually not trigger foods; it is not likely that someone will not be able to control their intake of acorn squash. Nonetheless, be aware of their carbohydrate and sugar content, and choose a variety of vegetables to eat that fit well with your diet plan.

You may have already heard that potatoes, sweet potatoes, and yams are rich in carbohydrates. Remember, potatoes come in many forms. French fries, hash browns, baked potatoes, boiled potatoes, and potato salads are all forms of potato. These classic starchy vegetables provide, on average, as many carbohydrates per serving as breads, cereals, and grains, though not as much protein as legumes and starchy beans. So, these should be avoided, as should their close relatives, parsnips and rutabagas, which are carbohydrate-rich root vegetables. It's hard to imagine anyone complaining about having to restrict their intake of rutabagas, but as mentioned earlier, potatoes are often used as side dishes for entrées, both at restaurants and at home. Knowing this, it's important to plan ahead so that you have healthy substitutions. So, what are your alternatives? There are so many different vegetables out there that your options are really almost endless. Vegetables like broccoli, cauliflower, onions, and mushrooms all have very low sugar equivalencies and can be consumed on this diet.

FRUITS

The question of whether you can and should eat whole fruits is an important question and, among the various low-carbohydrate diet plans out there, often a point of contention. Fruit can be high in sugars, including fructose, which occurs naturally. However, there

VEGETABLE CARBOHYDRATE CONTENT

Low-Carb Vegetables

This list is arranged from lowest to highest carbohydrate counts, but all are nonstarchy and generally low in carbohydrates. (Serving size = 1 cup)

VEGETABLE	CARB CONTENT
Endive	1.7 g
Romaine lettuce	1.8 g
Mushrooms	2.3 g
Celery	3.6 g
Pumpkin	4.2 g
Cauliflower	5.3 g
Zucchini (cooked)	6.0 g
Spinach (boiled)	6.8 g
Tomatoes	7.0 g
Eggplant	8.6 g
Spaghetti squash	10.0 g
Broccoli	11.2 g
Onions	16.2 g

Starchy (High-Carb) Vegetables

The main vegetables to be avoided when reducing carbohydrates are the starchier and sweeter vegetables.

VEGETABLE	CARB CONTENT
Artichokes	18.8 g
Sweet potatoes	23.0 g
Butternut squash	24.1 g
Parsnips (boiled)	26.5 g
Potatoes (boiled and mashed)	29.0 g
Corn	31.7 g
Yams (cooked)	46.0 g

are a few reasons why fruits can be beneficial to you and should not be eliminated.

First, as noted before, unlike other addictions, like heroin or alcohol, in which you can totally eliminate the substance from your life and never consume it again, it is practically impossible to do that with sugars. The goal of this plan is to reduce your dependence on them and to renegotiate the role they play in your life so that they're no longer used as a primary source of your pleasure and calories. So, if you need to consume some sugars, fruits are the best option.

This is because fruits might have sugar in them, but they also have a lot of nutritional value, and often contain antioxidants and other phytonutrients that are beneficial to our overall health. They also have a lot of fiber, so they will make you feel full after consuming them. Try to eat one to two pieces of fruit each day, and strive for fruits that have a low sugar equivalency. Blackberries, strawberries, and raspberries all have sugar equivalency values below 6, but raisins have a sugar equivalency of 71! Dried or dehydrated fruits, like raisins, are basically whole fruits with the water removed, and as a result, they end up being smaller in size, and thus have a higher ratio of sugar content. They tend to be better than fruit juices, in that they retain the fiber and nutrients that you get with whole fruits; however, sugar is often added to dehydrated fruits, so be sure to

SUGAR EQUIVALENCY OF FRUIT

Fruit	Per 100 Grams of Fruit	Fruit	Per 100 Grams of Fruit
Raisins	71	Pineapples	11
Dehydrated prunes	67	Tangerines	11
Dried apricots	55	Plums	10
Bananas	18	Apricots	9
Grapes	17	Oranges	9
Figs	16	Papayas	9
Cherries (sweet)	14	Peaches	8
Mangos	14	Grapefruits	7
Blueberries	12	Lemons or limes	6
Pears	12	Blackberries	5
Apples	11	Raspberries	5
Kiwifruits	11	Strawberries	5

inspect the nutrition labels. Plus, they are usually easier to eat than fresh fruit, and you may end up consuming more fruit in the dried form than you would otherwise. So, even though we typically think of fruit as being very healthy, it's a good idea to look up some of your favorite fruits in the Sugar Equivalency Table (see the box opposite) to get a better sense of which work well with this diet and which you can replace with other, less sugary options.

PROTEIN

Another large portion of your diet when reducing carbohydrates and sugars will consist of meat, poultry, and seafood, as almost all of these have a sugar equivalency of 0. As mentioned earlier, protein can be especially helpful when trying to lose weight, as it is very satisfying. In addition to being filling, the options with protein are seemingly endless, ensuring that your diet never gets boring. Chicken, turkey, beef, pork, ham, salmon, tuna, shrimp—the list goes on—and each of these can be prepared in different ways (for example, grilled, baked, sautéed) with countless different spices and seasonings. Meat and seafood can be used as warm salad toppings or can be stuffed with cheeses and vegetables for a more substantial entrée. You can also melt cheese on top of a serving of meat. Meat and cheese roll-ups are a great option for a quick, fulfilling snack, and meat and vegetable skewers are perfect for a summer barbeque. In addition to meat, poultry, and seafood, there are several other high-protein foods, including milk, cheese, eggs, yogurt, nuts, beans, soy products, and seeds; however, with these items, be sure to check to see how many carbohydrates or how much sugar they contain as these will vary.

Replacing the Taste that Comes with Hidden Sugars

Hidden sugars, or sugars that appear in foods where you would least expect to find them—like sauces, condiments, and dressings—are added to jazz up the taste. Since most sauces and condiments will be off-limits on this plan, what can you do to give a little extra pizzazz to your meal?

Spices can be used in place of sugar-containing condiments (such as ketchup, many salad dressings, and barbecue sauces) to add extra flavor and excitement to your food. There are sugar-free alternatives to condiments, but be sure to read the label to make sure your condiment is really sugar-free. In a pinch, when you don't have a sugarless option, one tip is to start out by dipping your fork into the salad dressing and then using it to pick up a piece of lettuce when eating salad. This way, you'll not only avoid wasting dressing, but also get a mouthful of flavor while consuming less sugar in total with each bite. As you adjust, you will want to consider making other changes, such as seasoning your salad with freshly squeezed lemon or lime juice instead of dressing (this is particularly good when using arugula), or sprinkling some rosemary and thyme on top of your chicken to add flavor instead of using barbecue sauce or other bottled marinade. Create your own marinades by putting a piece of meat, fish, or chicken in a resealable plastic bag and adding your favorite spices and a small amount of olive oil. You may even want to add some fresh nuts to a sandwich in place of sugar-containing peanut butter for a similar taste and added crunch. You can also get sugar-free peanut butter (or make your own with a bag of peanuts and a food processor), or try different types of nut butters, such as almond butter.

Over time, as you reduce your intake of sugars, you may begin to notice that your sense of taste changes. There are a few reasons why this might happen. For one, when you eat foods drenched in sugar, other flavors are masked. For example, the sweet taste of frosted cereal can dominate your mouth while the subtle taste of the grains in the cereal is not easily detected. Also, sugars activate sweet-taste receptors in our mouths, and when we consume a diet high in added sugars, those receptors can become desensitized, and as a result you may feel like you need to eat more and more sugar in order to detect the sweet taste. Once you stop eating excess sugars, the receptors' sensitivity will change, and as a result, your perception of how sweet things taste will also change.

Typical Meals on the Sugar Freedom Plan

We thought it might be helpful to see examples of the kinds of foods you can eat broken down by meal (see the box on page 132). Given the variety of foods that you can eat on this diet and how creative you can be in experimenting with your own preferences, the numbers of meals you can create on your own are really limitless. Once you get started and begin to identify foods that are sensible alternatives to the sugar-rich foods you used to eat, you'll be well on your way to making appropriate and delicious food choices without much effort at all.

NEVER SKIP BREAKFAST

Your mother probably told you time and time again that breakfast was the most important meal of the day, but like most things other people tell us to do, if we don't understand why, we are less likely to do it. You may be used to a hectic morning routine that leaves little time for breakfast, or you may be used to exchanging a healthy

SAMPLE MEALS ON THE SUGAR FREEDOM PLAN

BREAKFAST
- Eggs
- Bacon
- Ham
- Sausage
- Omelets (add in ham, cheese, mushrooms, onions, tomatoes, avocado, salsa, sausage, black olives, bacon, salt, and pepper)
- Sugar-free yogurt
- Fruit in milk
- Cheese, sausage, ham roll-up

LUNCH
- Green salad (easy on the croutons), low-carbohydrate dressing, or oil and vinegar
- Meat and cheese salad—sausage, ham, mozzarella or Monterey Jack cheese, avocado, tomato, olive oil
- Crab salad (imitation crab for the cost conscious)—crab, celery and pepper wrapped in lettuce

- Egg salad (watch the mayo; it can have added sugar)
- Tuna salad
- Chicken salad
- Hamburgers (add in cheese, bacon, tomato, onions, lettuce, but no bun)
- Chicken lettuce wrap (use large leaves of iceberg lettuce as the wrap)
- Turkey lettuce wrap
- Peanut butter sandwich (using low-carb bread and peanut butter with no sugar added)
- Soups
- Chili

SNACKS
- Nuts
- Cheese and ham and sausage with mustard
- Peanut butter with celery
- Avocado
- One piece of fruit

DINNER
- Chicken
- Turkey
- Hamburgers (no bun)
- Meatloaf (without the breading)
- Ribs (with sugar-free barbecue sauce and sugar-free ketchup)
- Steaks
- All meats
- All game
- Broccoli
- Cauliflower
- Zucchini (with sprinkled Parmesan and butter)
- All fish
- Shellfish
- Shrimp
- Lobster with butter

DRINKS
- Water
- Sugar-free drink mix
- Sugar-free sodas
- Tea
- Coffee

breakfast for a few more minutes of sleep. Why make a change now? Why is breakfast the most important meal of the day? Well, for one, forgoing breakfast also means forgoing all of the nutrients that breakfast can provide. It's been shown, for example, that individuals who eat breakfast consume significantly more nutrients per day than those who skip it.[9] Eating breakfast has also been shown to enhance cognitive performance in adolescents, indicating how valuable it can be for mental functioning.[10] Some studies have also shown an association between not eating breakfast and a higher BMI[11, 12] as well as weight regain after dieting.[13]

When Americans tour Europe, they are typically surprised to see a breakfast buffet of cheese, sausage, and ham laid out with a few crackers. But these are good breakfast choices, with few or no carbohydrates (sans the crackers). Foods like pancakes, French toast, or waffles with lots of syrup on them are not good options. They are loaded with sugar and carbohydrates that will leave you wanting to eat more and more.

Before this diet, your breakfast may have looked like the unhealthy breakfast of many Americans: chocolate doughnuts, sugary cereal with milk, and or a bagel with cream cheese, and, of course, coffee (light, with lots of cream and sugar), maybe washed down with a big glass of orange or apple juice. Now, after reading about and understanding how much sugar these foods contain, you probably see why this was not a good way to start off your day. But after recalling the earlier discussion of addiction, it might make sense as to why people reach for these types of foods first thing in the morning after a period of deprivation from them (that is, while they were sleeping).

While you may have to say good-bye to chocolate doughnuts on this diet, there's no reason why you can't enjoy getting out of bed and having a delicious and filling breakfast. One of the keys to successfully implementing this diet is to eat meals regularly, which means no skipping breakfast! Several options are listed in the box on page 132.

One great option for breakfast is eggs, which are a natural source of protein and have no sugar or carbohydrates in them. Plus, they're inexpensive and they're filling. You're fine eating the whole egg. But, if you're concerned about your cholesterol, you might want to remove the yolk since that's where all of the cholesterol comes from. Another great thing about eggs is that they can be prepared in several different ways (scrambled, sunny-side up, and so on), so your routine doesn't have to get boring. You can create almost any omelet you can think of: just toss in your favorite low-sugar-equivalency items. Eggs can be a great way to start your day, and omelets are a good way to sneak in more vegetables.

Aside from eggs, there are lots of other options for breakfast. For instance, you can enjoy sugar-free yogurt, but be careful. Some fruit-flavored yogurts say they are sugar-free, but when you read the nutritional information you may find there's plenty of sugar in the fruit jam that's added to the plain yogurt to make it fruit-flavored. You can always buy plain yogurt and add in your own fruit. If you chop the fruit into small pieces, you will get added fiber and still make the yogurt taste sweet.

LUNCH AND DINNER

Lunch and dinner can be interchangeable. For one of these meals, it is always a good idea to have a big green salad. Some salad dressings are good options, but be sure to watch the labels as many often contain added sugars. Be extra wary of those that are labeled "fat-free," since these often contain excess sugar to make up for the taste that's lacking from leaving out the fat. You can always use olive oil and vinegar, and be sure to limit the croutons. One way to spice up your salad is to add a piece of chicken or meat to it (either on the side or chopped up on top).

If you like sandwiches, you have to get creative since bread is high in carbohydrates and often has added sugars in it. You can still enjoy a good chicken, turkey, pastrami, or ham sandwich, or even a BLT, but instead of using two whole pieces of bread, try making a half of a sandwich with normal portions of cold cuts, or using thin sandwich bread, which is lower in sugars than standard-size bread slices. There are also several low-carbohydrate wraps and breads on the market today that are lower in carbohydrates than traditional breads.

Most soups are fine to eat, though you should stay away from soups that have a lot of rice or macaroni in them. Chili is a heartier soup and can be a good option for lunch or dinner, but, interestingly, kidney beans have a high sugar equivalency, so opt for chili that is light on beans.

For entrées, you can eat chicken, turkey, meatloaf, spareribs, steaks, hamburgers (without the bun), or any game meat that you

What If You Are a Vegetarian?

If you are a vegetarian, there is some good news and some bad news. The good news is that you are probably already used to being creative with your diet and conscientious about ingredients, especially when it comes to dining out. The bad news is that because meats and seafood are generally considered a staple for those on low-carbohydrate diets, you may have to get a little more creative than usual when trying to implement this plan. Fortunately, by now you're probably accustomed to using other foods rich in protein, such as tofu, seitan, cheese, nuts, and beans. Note that while tofu and seitan generally have low amounts of carbohydrates, it is important to check the nutrition labels for carbohydrate and sugar content as this can vary from company to company.

Because you already incorporate a lot of vegetables into your diet, you'll certainly find that's to your advantage when implementing this plan. As mentioned earlier, salads are a great option for either lunch or dinner (remember to check the nutrition labels on salad dressings). Topping salads with cubed tofu can give them some protein content so they are more satisfying. Grilled portobello mushrooms are another great addition to salads. Eggs, quiches, and omelets can serve as great meals, and, as mentioned earlier, vegetables can easily be added to omelets as well as some cheese. Other options for vegetarians include some hummus (check the nutrition label as this may vary from company to company) and sugar-free peanut and other nut butters.

enjoy. You can spice them however you want, and you can even include gravies, but be careful because many store-bought gravies contain added sugars. There's enough fish, shrimp, lobster, and shellfish in the ocean that you could prepare a different fish meal every dinner for a year and never have the same meal twice.

This is just the beginning of an enormous, varied menu of wonderful meals that you can create. If you look at this plan as an opportunity to get creative and to experiment with different spices and ingredients, or if you see it as a challenge that requires you to think outside the box, you can really enjoy this way of eating, instead of focusing on the limitations that it may involve. So much of this way of eating and how successful you can be on it depends on how you conceptualize it, so embrace your creativity and accept the challenge of cooking wonderful, healthy, tasty meals for yourself—and your family!

SNACKS

Studies suggest that snacking can be a double-edged sword when it comes to our waistlines. On the one hand, we are almost constantly surrounded by images of food or opportunities to consume it. TV commercials, convenience stores on the ride home from work, vending machines, and food trucks on the corner—they all entice us to eat. This makes it easy for us to snack without realizing how many calories we're consuming, or to make a pit stop because it's convenient and we feel like eating something. Snacking is so commonplace today that over 27 percent of children's daily caloric intake comes from snacks.[14] In fact, the increase in the number of meals and snacking is one of two key factors (the other being increased portion sizes) contributing to the finding that from 1977–78 to 2003–06, the average daily caloric intake among American citizens increased from 1,803 to 2,374 calories; that's an increase of more than 570 calories![15]

Does this mean that we should eliminate snacks from our diets? No. The key is to snack on foods with high nutritional value and to eat them in reasonable amounts. Instead of popping open a soda or munching on chips until the bag is almost empty, you need to adopt a different tactic to satisfy your hunger. It's much better to eat fruits and vegetables, because they contain fiber and nutrients, than sugary foods and drinks. In fact, one study showed that participants who ate dried plums as a snack were much less likely to want to consume more food than participants who ate low-fat cookies.[16] Although the dried fruit contained sugar, it also contained fiber, which the cookies did not, and fiber is thought to promote satiety. Interestingly, participants given the low-fat cookies were also much more likely to want a sweet- or savory-tasting food after their snack than those who were given the dried plums, suggesting that what we eat may predispose us to want certain types of food.

It is fine to snack on this diet, but make sure that you don't graze on snacks all day long. You shouldn't "pre-eat." *Pre-eating* is a term used to describe when someone eats to avoid getting too hungry and overeating at a meal. It's important to learn the delicate balance of letting yourself get hungry so that you can learn to recognize the signs that your body gives you to indicate a need for calories but not letting yourself get so hungry that you eat whatever you can get your hands on. Many of the snacks that you presently consume might be high in sugars, and you may consume them not because you're hungry but because you feel compelled to eat sugar. Over time on this diet, you'll find that you're snacking less because you lose your cravings for those types of food.

Unfortunately, we usually need snacks when we are on the run, and most conveniently packaged snacks are terrible for us. Things that are easy to grab—like candy bars, granola bars, and bags of potato chips—are the worst kinds of snacks. If you're at home, you can easily and quickly prepare a healthy snack that fits much better with this diet. If you know you'll be on the road or need to eat at the office, prepare healthy food at home and bring it in ziplock bag or container. That enables you to avoid the desperate choice you might make when time is limited and your only options are processed foods.

Other ideal snacks are nuts like almonds or cashews. These don't have 0 sugar equivalencies, but they're low enough to be considered an acceptable snack. And if you go to any health food store, you'll see that they're now selling sugar-free peanut butter (which you can eat with carrot or celery sticks).

Another type of snack food to be wary of is bars. People often think they are making a healthy choice by ditching their cookies and instead grabbing trail mix bars, energy bars, and fruit bars. They sound healthier, but when you read the nutrition labels, especially the carbohydrate and sugar content, you'll see that they can be just as detrimental to your diet goals.

DESSERT

You may be wondering how dessert fits into this diet, but fear not. Not only is dessert possible on this diet, but it can also be delicious. You just need to reconceptualize what a dessert might look like. If you are accustomed to junk-food types of desserts, you can choose things like sugar-free Jell-O. Countless recipes can be found online for sugar-free desserts, including a recipe for sugar-free sugar cookies! However, you don't want to fall into the habit of eating desserts often. Desserts should be special treats, not eaten after every meal. Desserts should not dominate your diet. Even though they can be made sugar-free, they are still almost all empty calories.

❋

In this chapter and the last, we've introduced information to help you put this plan into practice. When you first begin to reduce or eliminate certain types of foods or drinks, however, you may encounter two problems: withdrawal and cravings. Without appropriate strategies to manage them, withdrawal and cravings can derail your best efforts to adopt a healthy, low-carbohydrate diet. In the next two chapters, we will discuss each of these in detail and offer several suggestions for dealing with them so that you can achieve your goals.

FOOD FOR THOUGHT

Think about what you commonly consume for each meal, snack, and beverage. If it contains a high amount of sugar, consider a possible replacement. It may be helpful to use the Sugar Equivalency Table (see the appendix) to determine (a) whether a food or drink needs to be replaced and (b) possible options that you may like.

- What do you eat for breakfast? What are possible replacements?
- What do you eat for lunch? What are possible replacements?
- What do you eat for dinner? What are possible replacements?
- What beverages do you drink? What are possible replacements?
- What snacks do you eat? What are possible replacements?

STEP 6

Managing Your Withdrawal

"I always think that I am one of the
millions and millions of people that
struggles with an addiction to food."

—CARNIE WILSON, SINGER

As you've already learned, there is scientific support for the idea that certain parts of our brain react to drugs and some foods in the same ways.[1] There is still some uncertainty about what that similarity actually means[2] in terms of understanding why we have a hard time controlling what we eat and keeping off unwanted, unhealthy, excess body weight, but that doesn't mean that food dependence and abuse isn't serious or valid. It's true that people aren't robbing liquor stores for money to buy Twinkies, nor are they getting fired for showing up to work with a box of doughnuts (in fact, those people are often well liked in the office). But people who have tried to quit overeating multiple times and failed because they can't seem to stop indulging in high-calorie, low-nutrition, palatable foods know how powerful this addiction can be.

The Power of Your Addiction

Food addiction is not socially taboo like most other types of addiction. You don't have to hide it. There aren't many social consequences to worry about. There is no need to steal money to fuel your addiction because junk food is cheap. Also, you don't have to hide your rituals for "using"; you can do it in the office, at your desk, or at the playground. It is okay to bring junk food to all of these places; in fact, people often welcome and encourage it. Think about how many times you have been in an office and seen a bowl of candy sitting on the receptionist's desk. Have you ever seen a bowl of those tiny liquor bottles that you are served on airplanes? Probably not.

Just because sugar addiction may not be recognized by society doesn't mean that addiction to food cannot have a power over you like a drug. Remember that just fifty years ago many people laughed at the thought that cigarettes might be addictive. Cigarettes were advertised on television just as sugar-rich foods are today. Beautiful models smoked in TV advertisements just as models today sip sugary beverages.

Unless you have experienced the power of addiction firsthand, it can be difficult to comprehend what an addictive substance or behavior can truly do to a person. And if you don't understand how powerful an addiction can be in controlling your behaviors and thought processes, it may be more difficult to stop. Addictions are as powerful as they are because they manage to interfere with the proper functioning of your thought and reasoning processes.[3]

Anyone who has known an alcoholic can relate to this point. Many have tried hundreds of times to quit drinking alcohol but have been unsuccessful. Some have even had such bad experiences with alcohol that they swore they would never drink again, but a few days later, they are back to the bottle. What goes wrong?

People often (falsely) presume that alcoholics or smokers or even people who are overweight have no willpower, but that isn't the case. They can have tremendous amounts of willpower when you look at other aspects of their lives. However, this willpower seems to weaken when they try to resist the substance they are addicted to.

Something else appears to be going on. You can't tell alcoholics that the reason they continued to drink, even after realizing it was bad for their health and career, was because it tasted good or made them feel good. Similarly, this isn't an adequate explanation for why some people continue to eat sugary foods after they gain weight, simply because the sugar tastes sweet and it's pleasurable to eat. No, for some people, there's something else driving this behavior.

After a certain point, what leads people to continue to consume the substance is not necessarily the pleasure derived from using it, but rather they may be using the substance to avoid the nasty side effects of quitting: withdrawal.

As you learned in Step 3, addiction is a cycle (see page 61). Let's use the potato chip phenomenon as an example. You might crave a potato chip, eat a handful, and move on with your day. Over time, however, you may find that it takes larger amounts of potato chips to satisfy an increasing tolerance to them. Additionally, many people who have been eating a diet that is rich in carbohydrates experience fairly profound withdrawal symptoms (such as headaches and irritability) when they go without carbohydrates for some time. Powerful cravings for junk foods, sometimes made worse by withdrawal-like symptoms, may lead us to want to eat more and more of the food, which can then lead to breaking a diet and overeating.

Most people who are addicted to things like alcohol generally need to cut them out of their lives in order to function properly. Most rehabilitation facilities and programs recommend that an alcoholic quit drinking alcohol permanently. One drink, or even cues associated with drinking, can activate the brain in an extremely powerful way, leading people to seek out more alcohol. However, this isn't possible with food. As discussed in the previous chapters, food cannot be abstained from or avoided completely, as we need it to survive. Our goal here isn't necessarily to eliminate all sugar from your diet, as this may prove impossible and unnecessary for most people. Instead, the goal is to reduce the major sources of sugar in your diet (for example, sugary items like soda, candy bars, and so on) and to try to keep your sugar intake at a low level, instead of the excessive amounts that may be more typically consumed.

During this process, you will likely encounter two problems: withdrawal and cravings. This chapter includes a discussion of what to expect during withdrawal and how to cope with withdrawal symptoms. These symptoms, if not approached proactively and with the right mind-set, may weaken your resolve to avoid eating certain foods. As mentioned earlier, identifying, acknowledging, and addressing the symptoms associated with withdrawal from sugars and other carbohydrates are important parts of the process of changing your diet.

What to Expect During Withdrawal

You are probably already familiar with the concept of withdrawal as it relates to drug addiction. During withdrawal from drugs or alcohol, unpleasant symptoms can emerge, ranging from muscle aches and irritability to tremors.[4] The discomfort that can come along with the withdrawal process may lead some people to take the drug again just to avoid or stop these effects from occurring. In fact, the current *Diagnostic and Statistical Manual* criteria for substance dependence defines withdrawal as either (1) the presence of withdrawal symptoms that are typical for the drug or (2) suppressing or preventing such effects by using the drug or a similar substance. So, withdrawal is not only characterized by the symptoms that emerge after quitting but also by efforts to prevent these potential symptoms from occurring.

This process, where someone might take a drug just to avoid the unpleasant effects of *not* taking it, is sometimes thought of within the context of what is called the opponent-process theory. According to this theory, drug addiction is the result of a pairing of pleasure and withdrawal symptoms. When a person first starts to use a drug or substance, there are high levels of pleasure and low levels of withdrawal symptoms. Over time, however, this balance changes; as the levels of pleasure from using the drug decrease, the levels of withdrawal symptoms increase. Because of this process, a person might be motivated to keep using the drug despite a lack of pleasure from it; instead, they use the drug or substance to avoid feeling lousy from *not* using it.

Symptoms of withdrawal have not only been observed during abstinence following drug use but also during abstinence from some types of palatable foods. Withdrawal symptoms from food addiction can be both physical and psychological in nature. Researchers reviewing the literature regarding humans addicted to refined foods, such as sugar-rich, processed foods, report evidence of withdrawal when people stop eating such foods. For example, participants reported eating sugary foods to combat negative emotional states, such as when they felt anxious, depressed, or tired.[5] Also, as mentioned in Step 3, controlled studies show that laboratory animals with a history of overeating sugar show both behavioral and

THE OPPONENT-PROCESS THEORY OF ADDICTION

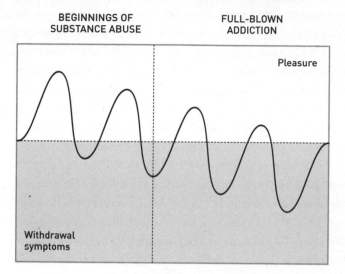

BEGINNINGS OF SUBSTANCE ABUSE

FULL-BLOWN ADDICTION

Pleasure

Withdrawal symptoms

neurochemical symptoms of withdrawal when sugar is no longer made available to them for a period of time. Tremors, teeth chattering, and higher levels of anxiety have all been observed in these animals, suggesting a state of withdrawal.[6]

As you begin to cut sugar and other carbohydrate-rich foods out of your diet, you may experience any of the following typical withdrawal symptoms:

- Fatigue
- Irritability
- Sadness
- Lethargy, lack of interest in exercise
- Headaches
- Strong cravings
- Drowsiness

Fortunately, withdrawal is an acute, or short, stage of the process. These feelings are not always apparent, but if they are, they usually subside within one to two weeks of changing the way that you eat. During this acute withdrawal phase when you first try to reduce your sugar intake, you may find yourself experiencing physical and or emotional symptoms, and your desire to consume these types of food may feel stronger. Try to remember that this compulsion to eat certain foods when abstaining from them is one of the main reasons people cheat when trying to follow some strict diet plans,[7] and may be why most diets end up failing.

If you find yourself becoming irritable, don't eat a sugary snack to make yourself feel better, and if you're tired, don't drink a sugar-filled soda to give a jolt to your blood sugar level. These feelings may be physical signs of withdrawal following a history of overconsuming sugar-rich foods. We've shared some strategies for dealing with the symptoms of withdrawal below, and as your body adapts, you'll feel more like your old self—and likely even better.

How to Manage Withdrawal Symptoms

If your mental image of withdrawal comes from the movies, you probably imagine intense sweats, trembling, and nausea. Those symptoms are more appropriate for a person quitting chronic drug use. Your symptoms, on the other hand, will probably be more subtle in nature. And if you follow our plan to gradually reduce your intake of sugars as outlined in Step 4, you will slowly taper down your intake, which means the withdrawal period may be less intense than if you quit eating all sugars cold turkey. However, it can be challenging in and of itself to make significant changes to your diet, and unpleasant symptoms such the ones listed above might lead you to want to throw in the towel altogether. So what can you do to counter the urge to consume sugar-rich foods if withdrawal symptoms emerge?

TIP 1: KEEP YOUR EYE ON THE LONG-TERM GAINS, NOT THE MOMENTARY PAINS

Remember that withdrawal is just a phase; it's one part of the addiction process. If unpleasant side effects of withdrawal begin and you feel like quitting, it's not your rational mind telling you to quit or your body telling you that you're denying it something that it needs. Instead, think of it as your addiction speaking, seeking to fulfill its urge.

Many times in our lives we have to sacrifice an immediate pleasure for rewards later on (for example, staying late at work to finish a project to put you in position for an upcoming promotion instead of meeting up with friends). However, if the rewards seem too far off, you may need to get a little creative in order to stay motivated. One technique that is often recommended to people who are trying to quit smoking may also be helpful for you: create a list, either in your mind or on paper, of your goals for implementing this plan.[8] Are you trying to lose weight before a major life event, like a wedding or high school reunion? Has your doctor told you that you need to change your diet for important health reasons? Do you find that you have less energy than you need to live an active and fulfilling life? Or maybe you're just tired of experiencing the highs and lows of a sugar-rich diet. Whatever your reasons are, get them clear in your mind or write them down so they are available as helpful and inspirational reminders when you encounter a problem. Remember, it's not worth it to quit just because of some temporary discomfort; the rewards are too great in the long run. The key is not to lose sight of these rewards during the day-to-day challenge of changing your diet.

TIP 2: ASK FOR SUPPORT

Evidence from addiction research has shown that social ties can be very important during recovery.[9, 10] For this reason, it's great to have the support of family and friends as you embark on this change in your diet. Although not everyone will identify themselves as food or sugar addicts, some of your friends or members of your family—to lose weight or for other health reasons—may want to join you as you reduce your sugar intake. Even if you can't find a friend or loved one to walk with you through all of the phases of the Sugar Freedom Plan outlined in Step 4 (see page 84), it may be helpful to talk to members of your family or friends about what you're doing and why so that they have the chance to support you. Telling people in your life that you may need their encouragement to stay on track with your health and eating goals will provide you with an extra bit of support, which may be especially helpful if you find yourself wavering on your decision to make healthy changes during withdrawal. It will also give them forewarning that you might be in a bad mood for a little while. Remember, irritability has been noted when reducing carbohydrates and sugar.[11] Before you find yourself lashing out at your friends and family, it can be helpful to warn them.

Also, you may find that not everyone in your life is supportive of your new eating style. Some people may skeptically question your eating habits, tell you that you don't need to lose weight or change anything about yourself (even when you know that you do), or dismiss your new way of eating as silly or faddish. Remember that although you might feel like they are being unsupportive, they may actually be trying to make you feel good. One way to deal with this type of interaction is to say, "Thanks. I know you always see the best in me no matter what, but I really want to make some changes in my diet and lifestyle, so it would be great if you could support me and be understanding of my decisions." On the other hand, some people you may interact with might be downright rude and dismissive of your new eating habits. If you encounter someone like this, you can try to explain to her why you are eating this way and what you have learned about addiction and food from this book. If she still isn't convinced, then just end the conversation and move on to a new discussion. You don't need to justify yourself to anyone, so if she isn't interested in being serious about something that is important to you, just don't talk to her about it. There are plenty of other people in your life whom you can lean on for support.

TIP 3: HOPE FOR THE BEST, BUT PLAN FOR THE WORST

Although this section of the book may seem like a forecast for doom and gloom, it isn't designed to scare you. If you're aware of the potential signs and symptoms of withdrawal that may emerge, you can use this knowledge to avoid falling back into an addictive eating trap in an effort to make yourself "feel better." If we apply what we know about addiction using the opponent-process model (which is the method by which pleasant feelings associated with an action gradually diminish and are taken over by negative feelings, such as withdrawal), it is possible to find yourself eating foods that you know you should avoid just to alleviate the negative feelings that you experience during withdrawal. If you're aware that this may happen, you can make a conscious effort not to act on these impulses to eat if they arise.

Not everyone experiences withdrawal. So, you may not even experience symptoms of withdrawal, or they may emerge in the form of subtle inconveniences. Just as withdrawal symptoms may be different in nature and more or less severe from one person to another, certain coping mechanisms may be more or less effective for different people during this period. Some people may find it more helpful than others to call up a friend and share how they're feeling. Others may find it more helpful to go to the range and hit golf balls or get crafty and begin a new project. Tailor your strategy for coping with withdrawal symptoms to what you're comfortable with and what works for you. Whatever it is that you do, just know that these negative feelings will pass.

It may be helpful to think about and plan for techniques that appeal to you *before* you begin to experience withdrawal symptoms so you'll be prepared if they emerge. You don't want to find yourself defenseless if or when these feelings arise. Take a moment to think about how you typically handle unpleasant situations, whether they are characterized by negative emotional states or physical symptoms like headaches, and whether these methods have been effective for you in the past. Have a plan (or two) in place for how you can react if you get a craving for a food or if you are feeling bad. Instead of reaching for a cookie, grab a crunchy, healthy snack (like a handful of almonds or a few carrots) or go for a quick walk around the block. If you're feeling irritable, maybe a relaxing soak in the tub or an afternoon working in the garden would calm you down. Play a game with your children, clean out the hall closet, or settle down on the couch with that article that you've wanted to read. Try a new workout class at the gym, go to a movie, or meet some friends for coffee. Could any of these techniques be used if you find yourself experiencing withdrawal symptoms? If not, what might work for you?

Finally, don't beat yourself up if you backslide a little and have a piece of chocolate after dinner one night or grab a can of soda when there is nothing else available. Don't let these little slipups derail your whole diet. You can always wake up tomorrow with a renewed sense of dedication to changing to your diet.

✳

Remember, withdrawal is an acute stage, not a constant struggle. The goal is to make it successfully through this stage without falling back into unhealthy eating habits. Unfortunately, there is no "cure" for withdrawal—there is nothing that you can do to prevent it from happening (aside from not getting dependent on certain foods in the first place). Keeping your goals in the forefront of your mind, keeping your friends and family members close, and being prepared with coping mechanisms that work for you are all strategies that may make navigating this period a little bit easier. A quote from a book entitled *The Adversity Paradox*, by J. Barry Griswell and Bob Jennings, describes another key point to remember when considering the process of withdrawal: "Adversity is never the end point; for those faced with a positive attitude, it's always the beginning."[12] Though withdrawal may be unpleasant at times, it may also mark the beginning of the end of an addiction.

Along with or independent of withdrawal, you may experience cravings for the foods that you are reducing or eliminating. The following chapter is designed specifically to help you address and

FOOD FOR THOUGHT

- Why are you implementing the Sugar Freedom Plan?

- Why is this important to you?

- What two techniques can you use to manage withdrawal symptoms if they arise? For example, if you're feeling irritable on the third day without your normal sugar fixes, what might help to turn your mood around?

STEP 7

Managing Your Cravings

"The belly rules the mind."

—SPANISH PROVERB

Cravings are normal, extremely common events. Most people can identify a time when they craved a food. You can crave foods that you don't end up eating, and you can eat foods that you don't crave. Craving can be considered on a continuum of experiences that range from mild to extreme. While it is part of the normal appetitive process, when it comes to addiction, cravings can seem out of control and become all-consuming.

Food cravings have a two-part definition: (1) they require a strong urge, and (2) they require that that urge be directed toward eating a specific food item.[1] This separates a craving from hunger, which may motivate a person to eat anything. Many people falsely mistake specific food cravings for hunger. Some rationalize that when you crave a piece of cake, it is your body's way of telling you that you are hungry and need to eat. In fact, this is the opposite of what the science tells us. For example, a recent controlled study found that when participants were hungry, food cravings actually went *down*.[2] Even when people are on long-term, low-calorie diets to induce weight loss, they report fewer cravings and claim to be less hungry.[3]

However, there is a difference between hunger and dieting. In the studies discussed above, the people were hungry, meaning that they were fasting or were on a very low-calorie diet; they were in a state of caloric need. If they are on appropriate diets, dieters usually aren't experiencing a caloric deficit. Instead, they eat the right amount of calories, but they eat healthier foods than they might be used to. A recent study found that when dieters are asked about their cravings, they report increased thoughts about their craved foods or feeling strong urges to eat, and these cravings are reported to be significantly stronger and more difficult to resist and to linger in dieters compared to those who are not actively dieting.[4] Unfortunately, the phrase "absence makes the heart grow fonder" may not just apply to romance but also to your diet. So, when trying to reduce your sugar intake, you may find yourself craving sugar-rich foods.

It should be noted, however, that over the years, mixed evidence has accumulated regarding whether people are more likely to experience cravings while hungry, dieting or not. It may be that food cravings are more likely for some people than others. Individuals with an addiction to food may be especially accustomed to experiencing cravings for food, and when certain foods are restricted, these cravings may feel even stronger. At times, urges to eat certain foods can feel irresistible, and they can consume your thoughts and behaviors. But here is the good news: while cravings may arise when making any change in the way you eat, especially when giving up foods that may be involved in an addictive cycle, (1) cravings are acute episodes, which will pass, (2) resisting them is (probably not surprisingly) associated with improved weight loss,[5] and (3) you can take steps to reduce the intensity and incidence of these cravings.

You might wonder if these cravings will last or if they will continue to be as strong as they may seem at first. Fortunately, research has been able to lend some insight into this as well. A study comparing a low-carbohydrate diet to a low-fat diet found that participants assigned to the low-carbohydrate diet showed a more significant reduction in carbohydrate cravings.[6] This reduction was apparent three months following the start of the diet and was further reduced at twelve months. Additionally, participants assigned to the low-carbohydrate diet reported a reduced preference for foods rich in carbohydrates and sweets compared to those assigned to the low-fat diet. Cravings for sugar were also decreased by three months, although after three months, these increased, suggesting the importance of using craving avoidance techniques, a few of which will be discussed next, even as time goes on. These results indicate that cravings for both carbohydrates and sugar can decrease even within the first three months.

Junk Food Consumption

Between the 1970s and 1990s, frozen potato consumption rose 63 percent based on reports from the US Department of Agriculture, evidence of a dramatic rise in french fry consumption.[7] Also, estimates of the amounts of particular junk foods consumed by Americans yearly, per person, are alarming: 50 pounds of cookies and cakes, 100 pounds of refined sugar, 55 pounds of fat and oil, 300 containers of soda, 20 gallons of ice cream, 5 pounds of potato chips, and 18 pounds of candy![8]

Food cravings can be a major obstacle to weight-loss success. In fact, researchers have found that the number one reason people reported not entirely following a strict diet during certain feeding studies was that they experienced food cravings.[9] Because of the powerful effect that cravings can have on our food-intake patterns, it is important to have an arsenal of strategies on hand to avoid giving in to them if they arise.

Combating Your Cravings

While withdrawal is normally an acute phase that will eventually pass, cravings for certain foods may linger. This is because, as noted above, craving is a part of the normal appetitive process, and also because cues, situations, or memories of foods that you used to over-consume can arise at any time and perhaps weaken your resolve. Here are some pointers on how you can tame your cravings to stay on track with your healthy eating habits.

UNDERSTAND WHAT YOU CRAVE

The category of junk food is composed of those things that we know we aren't supposed to eat too much of, but we eat them anyway: chips, ice cream, cake, cookies, chocolate bars, and so on. These processed foods are usually very high in calories and very low in nutritional value. Americans seem to spend a lot of time in the junk food aisles of the grocery store because, as a nation, we consume a lot of junk food. Factors such as low cost, convenience, and habit are all to blame, and as you are learning, addiction may also explain in part why people like to eat these particular foods so much and in such large quantities. Most junk foods contain a lot of added sugars.

HEALTHIER SUBSTITUTES FOR CRAVED FOODS

TYPE OF JUNK FOOD	CHARACTERISTIC YOU CRAVE	ALTERNATIVES
Chips	Crunchy	Carrots, celery, any vegetable paired with hummus or peanut butter
Chocolate	Sweet	Fruit
Cookies	Sweet and crunchy	Apple slices with low-fat string cheese
Ice cream	Sweet and creamy	Frozen fruit smoothie with black tea and mint
Pretzels	Crunchy and salty	Lightly salted nuts or seeds
Soda	Carbonation or fizz	Seltzer, mineral water
Sugary candy	Sweet	Sugar-free Jell-O, fresh raspberries

It is reported that, on average, Americans consumed 152 pounds of added sugars in 2000.[10] In fact, in 2000, daily consumption of added sugars amounted to approximately 32 teaspoons for each person, which is about three times higher than the limit recommended by the USDA.[11] So not only is junk food bad for you because of the added calories and lack of nutrients, but if it is loaded with sugar, it may fuel your addiction and lead you to want to continue to eat these foods, which will definitely pack on the pounds.

When initiating any change in your eating habits, by and large, junk foods are the largest class of foods that needs to be eliminated (see Eliminate Junk Foods, page 102); however, they can also be the hardest to give up. But there are alternatives to junk food. The key is to identify *what* it is about the food that you crave, and then try to substitute it with a more appropriate food. For example, if you crave potato chips, think about what aspect of the chip you want to eat. Is it because you want something salty? Something crunchy? The table above outlines some commonly craved categories of junk foods and offers some healthier substitutions based on their qualities. It is simply a matter of finding the alternative food that will satisfy you, at least enough to get you through the acute period in which you crave that particular food.

UNDERSTAND WHEN AND WHY YOU CRAVE

Some research has focused on how our emotional state may influence food cravings. On a regular (often daily) basis, people may feel stressed as a result of their jobs, families, or uncertainties about the future. There is evidence that when people are stressed, they increase the amounts of sugar and fat-rich foods they eat.[12] This is related to the finding that stress stimulates the release of cortisol, a steroid hormone, which has been shown to stimulate appetite.[13]

Food, and in particular comfort foods, or highly palatable foods, may make us feel better. This could be for a number of reasons. For instance, it has been suggested that we may feel better because these foods give us some sense of pleasure, and eating them may serve as a distraction from stress or may moderate our stress response.[14, 15, 16] All of these possibilities may help to explain why some people turn to food to cope with difficult situations in their lives. However, the types of food that people seem to turn to during these times generally are not healthy options. For instance, one study found that psychological distress among women was associated with food cravings for sweets and fast food.[17] Another study among college women found that about 60 percent of participants reported an increased appetite when stressed, but only 33 percent reported eating healthy foods when stressed (versus 80 percent when not stressed). Instead, when stressed, participants tended to consume sweets and mixed dishes such as pizza or fast food.[18]

Using food as a coping mechanism is not a healthy approach to dealing with stress or unpleasant emotions, especially considering the possible consequences of weight gain and other health concerns like diabetes. So, if you find that you often crave food when things in your life seem stressful, consider other, healthier coping mechanisms that might serve a similar function to eating. The key is to identify what function eating serves for you in that moment. Is it a temporary distraction? Does it make you feel better? Similar to junk food, you can find a healthier substitution depending on how you think it benefits you. For example, if it serves as a distraction, what else might work instead? Taking the dog for a walk? Reading a book? Listening to music? The alternative is entirely up to you and based on your needs, which may vary depending on the situation.

Variety Is the Spice of Life

Recent research using brain-imaging techniques has tried to investigate the effects of food craving on our brains. One study found that certain areas of the brain showed increased activation when participants thought about foods they enjoy.[19] These brain areas, the researchers note, overlap with some brain regions associated with drug craving. What is particularly interesting about this study is that it was only participants who were placed on a monotonous or boring diet—that is, a diet that lacked variety—who showed increased activation in these brain regions when they thought about the food items they like. These findings again suggest common neural mechanisms related to both palatable foods and drugs, but also that the assortment of foods we eat may influence how strong a craving may be. They also emphasize the need to have an array of recipes and different foods on hand so that your meals don't become too mundane.

Be Aware of Food Cues

We encounter environmental food cues almost everywhere we look, and the effects of these food cues may have a subtle but powerful influence on our decisions regarding what to eat. Food packaging, labels, logos, commercials, catchy songs—all serve to remind us of the enjoyable experience of eating certain foods in the hopes that we will buy and eat more of them. It's Marketing 101. And the worst part is that we seem to live in a society that is one big food cue. Unfortunately, there are very few cues to eat kale or celery sticks.

Cues can be visual, mental, auditory, or even olfactory (smelled). So, if you get the hankering for a can of soda while watching a movie, it may be the result of a cleverly placed product that is serving as a cue. If you get an urge to eat apple pie when you get to Grandma's house, it may be your surroundings acting as a mental cue of the many pies that she has baked for you in the past. If you hear the music of the ice-cream truck coming down the road, you might suddenly be dying for a cone. If you are trying to cut down on sugar- and carbohydrate-rich foods, it's important to recognize these powerful cues so that you can minimize the effect they may have on your food choices.

Let's say you're driving on the highway and see the logo of your favorite fast-food chain. You suddenly sense an urge to consume a certain food or drink from that place and decide to go there. This behavior is a typical example of classical conditioning. Classical conditioning is a learning technique first discovered by Ivan Pavlov, who is best known for his work conditioning dogs. Classical conditioning involves an unconditioned stimulus, unconditioned response, neutral stimulus, and conditioned response. An unconditioned stimulus triggers an unconditioned response naturally; it does not need to be learned. For instance, if you smell your favorite food and then find yourself feeling hungry, the food's flavor is serving as the unconditioned stimulus and your feeling of hunger is the unconditioned response. During classical conditioning, an unconditioned stimulus is associated with a neutral stimulus so that the neutral stimulus is able to elicit the unconditioned response, which is then called the conditioned response because it has been learned.

This is what happens when we see a food logo. We have become conditioned such that when we see the neutral stimulus of a logo (which is merely an image with which we associate meaning), we feel the urge to consume some food or drink. This is why when you see the McDonald's arches, you can almost taste the french fries, and you may suddenly want to stop in and get some even if you aren't hungry. This is also why McDonald's has had the same basic logo since the company's inception and has it advertised in as many places as it can: the arches are a cue that signals the availability of french fries. In fact, we are so programmed to want to obtain this

HOW CLASSICAL CONDITIONING WORKS

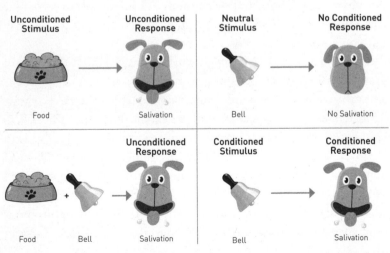

food reward that when we see the food cue, we anticipate the pleasure of eating. This anticipation helps to reinforce this association and behavior.

As a side note related to fast-food logos, there is evidence that children recognize these logos at a higher frequency than other food logos,[20] and scientists suggest that this increased recognition could lead children to influence their parents' buying behaviors.[21]

Numerous studies have also shown the effect that certain cues can have on our brains. Scientists have found that cues associated with drug use can elicit similar neurochemical responses as actual drug use. For instance, in rats, it has been shown that just being exposed to stimuli related to previous cocaine use can result in a release of dopamine in the brain,[22] and in humans, heightened neural activation in reward-related brain regions is seen in human drug addicts who are shown drug cues, like heroin paraphernalia.[23]

HOW FOOD-CUE CONDITIONING WORKS

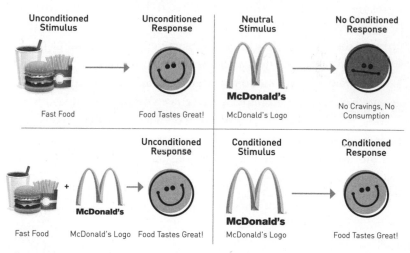

Interestingly, studies reveal that people who are obese show stronger neural activation in response to food cues and seem to exert more effort to control their appetite when encountering these cues.[24] People who are overweight also tend to view pictures of food more readily than lean people, especially when they report having a food craving. Thus, when experiencing a food craving, an individual who is overweight may have a heightened awareness of the food cues around him. Being overweight has also been associated with greater snack food intake after viewing food cues than healthy-weight controls.[25] Cues do their job: they make us want to eat foods. And unfortunately, if you are overweight or obese, they may be even more effective.

So what can we do to control any programmed response we may have when we see, smell, hear, or are reminded of such food cues? The first and most important step is to recognize what these cues are doing. The second step is to recognize what *you* need, or do not need, to eat or drink in that moment. By being mindful of your own needs, instead of what corporations may try to encourage you to eat, you can make smart decisions regarding your diet despite exposure to food cues. Would you agree to buy something from a telemarketer who calls you persistently, even if you did not need the product they were selling? No. The same concept applies to food stimuli and rewards. With a telemarketer, you evaluate what you have and realize that you do not need what he is trying to sell you, despite his incessant attempts to convince you that you do, so you decline, hang up the phone, and move on with your day. Likewise, with food cues, you can move past them or change the channel and continue to stay on track with your long-term goals.

Have a Plan

As mentioned in Step 6, strategies that are recommended to help people successfully cope with cigarette cravings when trying to quit smoking may also be helpful when conquering an addiction to sugar, and especially when trying to avoid cravings for certain foods.[26] These include setting a time frame, such as fifteen minutes, when you first get a craving. Try to go for fifteen minutes without indulging the craving. At the fifteen-minute point, your craving may be less strong and easier to avoid, or you may have become engaged in or distracted by something else and forgotten about it altogether. If you experience a craving, it may be helpful again to list and reflect upon your long-term goals: why you are not indulging in these foods. Try to keep these long-term goals in mind when you find yourself craving an unhealthy food that will probably only satisfy you temporarily and, in the long run, may maintain a cycle of addiction.

✳

When trying to conquer an addiction to sugar, cravings may threaten to hinder progress and long-term success. With a better understanding of what contributes to our cravings, however, we're better prepared to handle them more effectively. This chapter has emphasized the importance of understanding why you crave certain foods versus others, when you tend to crave these foods, the influence of food cues in eliciting cravings, and the importance of variety when it comes to cravings. With this information and some of the suggestions included above, you should be better able to handle these cravings if they arise.

FOOD FOR THOUGHT

- Are there any foods or drinks that you commonly crave?

- What is it about these foods or drinks that you find appealing or appetizing?

- Knowing this, what are some healthier foods or drinks that you may be able to use as substitutions? (You may want to use the Sugar Equivalency Table in the appendix as a guide.)

- Do you find that you tend to crave foods or drinks in certain circumstances (for example, when you are stressed, sad, or excited)? Aside from eating, how else might you respond to or cope with these situations or moods when they arise?

STEP 8

Avoiding a Relapse (and What to Do If One Occurs)

> *"Always bear in mind that your own resolution to success is more important than any other one thing."*
>
> —ABRAHAM LINCOLN

For some people, this might be the most important chapter in this book. Maybe you've been excited and committed to starting other diets before, but one poor food choice, one slipup that you regretted the minute you made it, left you feeling disappointed in yourself and discouraged about your ability to stick to a diet plan, and ultimately derailed you from continuing. This process of events—eating a certain food or more food than planned, which leads to negative thoughts and emotions (such as frustration, disappointment, and guilt), which leads to throwing in the towel—is precisely what this chapter has been designed to help safeguard against.

First, let's briefly describe how a *relapse* is defined. As mentioned in earlier chapters, sugars and other carbohydrate-rich foods are almost everywhere. In fact, they are even contained in many drinks and food items that people often consider healthy options (such as dried fruit, trail mixes, and protein or granola bars), so totally eliminating sugar from your diet would be nearly impossible. The goal of this plan is to eliminate the major sources of excess added sugars and other carbohydrates from your diet, such as sugary beverages and junk foods like candy bars and various desserts, as a way to reduce your overall sugar intake. So it isn't as though if you consume some sugar you are relapsing or breaking the rules of this plan; consumption of a high amount of sugar, however, would constitute a regression, and if this continued over a longer period of time, this would constitute a relapse.

Before discussing what to do if a relapse occurs, it's important to talk about some factors that can aid in preventing a relapse from occurring in the first place. The withdrawal symptoms and cravings discussed in Steps 6 and 7 represent possible risk factors for relapsing, but hopefully with the information covered in those chapters, you are better equipped to handle these challenges. Understanding the process and some of the symptoms associated with withdrawal can help you to identify and contextualize them as temporary indications that your body is adjusting to a new way of eating. Additionally, having an awareness of the types of foods you tend to crave, when you tend to crave them, and what function they serve for you can help you to develop alternative strategies that do not include giving in to food cravings. The concept of food cues has also been discussed in previous chapters, and it is important to be aware of these and to be confident about how you can handle them, as they may also contribute to a relapse. In this chapter, several other factors that may be associated with relapse will be discussed.

Make Sure That You Are Thinking Straight

Studies assessing predictors of weight regain following a diet provide a wealth of information regarding the factors that may contribute to a relapse. Studies show dichotomous thinking to be the number one difference between participants who regained weight they had lost after one year and those who kept it off.[1] You're probably wondering, What in the world is dichotomous thinking, and *do I do it*?

Dichotomous thinking can be described as black-and-white thinking or thinking in extremes. Suppose someone received a poor grade on a history test. That person might think, "I did poorly on that test. Maybe I didn't study enough or maybe history isn't my thing." Someone using dichotomous thinking, on the other hand, might conclude, "I'm not smart." You can easily see how this kind of extreme thinking can get you into trouble when it comes to food-intake behaviors. Maybe someone who has been trying for a few weeks to lose weight eats one piece of candy and then thinks, "Forget it! I just cheated and messed up my diet. I might as well eat the whole bag now." It's this kind of thinking that can lead to a regression or relapse and perhaps even to giving up altogether. Therefore, it's very important to think about how you will handle situations like this ahead of time and to develop strategies for yourself to avoid dichotomous or black-and-white thinking. One helpful technique in this type of situation may be to think about the consequences before you act. Take a moment to think about how you will feel if, after eating something you were avoiding, you (a) choose to stop and reassess the situation calmly or (b) choose to adopt black-and-white thinking and spiral into a binge. How will you feel afterward if you choose option a? How about if you choose option b?

Keep Tabs on Your Emotions, and Cope Accordingly

Another study investigating the factors associated with weight regain found that participants with a tendency to eat when they thought or felt negative thoughts or emotions showed less weight loss at six- and eighteen-month follow-ups.[2] These participants were considered to have their eating influenced more by internal than external stimuli. This finding can be helpful in two ways.

First, it brings us back to the discussion in Step 7 about the importance of identifying the situations in which you may find yourself craving foods. Do you find yourself eating certain foods or eating more when you are depressed or stressed (examples of internal stimuli), or when you are in certain situations, like at a work event (an example of an external stimuli)? Once you identify when and why you tend to eat certain foods or overeat, you can then brainstorm other ways to handle these situations that don't involve compromising your diet goals. For example, if you find that you are yearning for certain foods in an attempt to alleviate anxiety or depression (either internally or as a result of an external stressor), tell yourself that you are not hungry and don't need to eat, and instead do something else to distract your feelings: go for a walk, see if the mail arrived yet, check your email, and so on. Do something to change your environment. If that doesn't seem to do the trick and you are still feeling like you need food to make you feel better, then you need to find a more healthy coping behavior. Instead of reaching for a carbohydrate-rich snack when you are feeling blue, maybe you can work on an art project, clean your house, or do some gardening. Choose something that you enjoy (yes, even housework can be rewarding for some of us!), and draw your happiness from an activity other than eating.

Significant differences have also been noted between individuals who regained the weight they had lost and those who kept the weight off in terms of the different types of coping behaviors they used when encountering stress or issues in their lives.[3] Those who kept the weight off reported using more problem-solving and problem-confronting strategies (for example, asking someone for help with a difficult project or discussing how they felt with someone who had upset them), whereas those who gained the weight back reported using more escape and avoidance techniques, such as eating, sleeping, and so on.[4] These responses represent two very different ways of coping with problems that may have implications for following a diet.

Another interesting line of thinking suggests that relapse prevention should not only focus on avoiding negative patterns of behavior but also on creating and emphasizing positive ones.[5] For example, doing things like starting a new hobby, expanding your social life, or simply doing more things you find to be fun may actually be beneficial to your diet. Compared to people who regained the weight they lost, people who kept the weight off during the next year reported spending more time relaxing or doing what they find pleasurable, as well as spending more time on work.[6] This finding suggests the importance of other parts of your life, aside from the ones that people often think of when dieting (eating, exercising, and so on). Although concentrating on other aspects of your life may not directly help you to lose weight, doing so may help protect you against stressors and cues that can contribute to weight regain.

Have a Diet That's Tailor-Made

Researchers have also reported that the perspective and approach one takes when implementing a diet plan appears to differentiate individuals who keep lost weight off and those who gain it back. For example, one group of researchers has reported that participants who identified themselves as "maintainers" were more likely to have tailored their diet plans to their lifestyle, whereas those participants who identified themselves as "relapsers" seemed to go to more drastic extremes (by fasting, having certain diet foods, and so on).[7] This finding suggests that in order to be most effective, these changes should be sustainable, meaning that you can keep doing them over the long run. There is no one-size-fits-all approach when it comes to dieting; take what you learn and adapt it to your life in ways that work for *you*. That is one of the advantages of this diet plan: you can change it to fit your lifestyle, and you can continue to adapt it over time as your needs and circumstances change.

This group of researchers also pointed out another important difference between the two groups: those who regained weight reported feeling deprived when dieting, while the maintainers tried not to.[8] What are some ways that you can stick to this diet without feeling like you're missing out? This may require experimenting with some different ingredients and recipes to figure out ways to make and enjoy delicious foods.

Remember Your Goals, and Revise Them as Needed

You probably know all too well that one of the most difficult things to face is weight regain. It is sad when you have been at, or close to, your weight-loss goals, and then something goes awry that leads you to fall back into old eating habits. This "something" could be many things, including that the diet really didn't fit with your lifestyle or it wasn't realistic. Or, maybe you viewed the diet as a temporary situation and you thought you could go back to your old eating habits once you lost a bit of weight.

However, another factor can play a significant part in weight regain: not having a clear, realistic goal in place, or losing sight of one's goals, which minimizes their importance. In one study, participants who lost weight were asked about their priorities regarding maintaining their weight loss; those who regained weight in a year after losing it reported weight control as less of a priority than participants who kept the weight off.[9] This finding indicates the importance of how much we value our goals. If you get to a point where you're happy with your body weight and have met your goals, congratulations! At this point, it is time to reset your goals, perhaps to focus instead on maintaining a certain weight loss for a certain time period. Avoid setting goals that are too vague or undefined (for example, "I will stay this weight forever"). Instead, give yourself incremental goals (such as, "I will not gain any weight back over the next two weeks") that you can work toward and be encouraged by your continued successes when you achieve them.

What to Do if You Regress or a Relapse Occurs

First, take a deep breath. It's not the end of the world. Try to reflect on all the progress you've made up until that point and remind yourself that one regression will not negate that progress. If you experience a full relapse—if you go back to your old eating habits and consume high amounts of sugar for several days, weeks, months, or longer—that's okay; you're still able to start fresh. Again, try not to use black-and-white thinking: you can be accountable for your mistakes while also feeling confident about your strengths and accomplishments. When you're in a relaxed state of mind, consider what factors may have contributed to the relapse. You will want to assess what happened from different angles, particularly how you were feeling, where you were, and any outside factors (such as an argument with a friend, a bad day at work, and so on) that could have contributed to your change in eating. Here are some questions that may be useful if you are reflecting on your relapse:

- Were you stressed?
- Were you experiencing feelings of self-doubt or apathy?
- In what kind of environment did your relapse occur? Were you attending a party or a holiday gathering?
- Was peer pressure a factor?
- When you were buying groceries, did you have a list? Were you hungry when you went to the store?
- How many hours of sleep were you getting in the nights preceding the relapse?

By understanding the factors that may have contributed to your relapse, you will be able to learn from your experience and apply this knowledge in a way that will help you stay on track in the future. Identify one or two specific factors that may have caused you to revert back to your old ways. Let's say you hadn't been getting much sleep, and then you went to a party where lots of sugar-rich foods were served and you deviated from your commitment to healthy eating habits. In this case, the two factors that contributed to the relapse were (1) your lack of sleep and (2) the food environment at the party. Choose one of these two factors and work to make sure that it won't be an issue if the situation arises again in the future. You might want to focus on making sure you get a certain number of hours of sleep per night or concentrate on putting together a balanced plate at the next party you attend. Regardless of why you relapsed, reflecting on the circumstances surrounding the relapse can allow you to see at least one thing that you can work on to avoid a relapse in the future.

Again, it's important to pay attention to how you think about your relapse. You can become guilt-ridden and think of it as an indication of failure, or you can take a more positive attitude and consider it an experience from which you can learn. This choice between assuming a positive or negative attitude toward the relapse may seem simple, but your attitude can be a powerful guide for your emotions, thoughts, and behaviors; your attitude can help you persist and succeed, or it can lead you to self-defeat. Your success depends on your commitment to assessing your behavior, learning from it, and making changes accordingly, even when you feel like giving up. Remember, with an understanding of why you may have relapsed, you will be better equipped to avoid another relapse in the future.

❋

It's a very delicate balance between understanding the power of addiction over your thought processes and behaviors, and being mindful of the role you play in the development and maintenance of, and the recovery from, the addiction. This means that you have to be honest with yourself, and with that comes admitting that you have a problem with some foods. Just like a drug addict or an alcoholic uses these drugs in a way that is out of control, you too may have to admit that foods serve as addictive substances and affect your mind and your ability to act in the ways that you desire. It is important that you acknowledge the power of the addiction process, but also know that you are not entirely powerless over it.

Here are some words of encouragement that you can tell yourself, especially when you are in a moment of weakness or on the brink of a relapse: "I can conquer addiction. I am stronger than the addiction. I can regain control over my food choices and body weight."

FOOD FOR THOUGHT

- Imagine that you have just gotten slightly off track after weeks of adhering to this new plan by eating something high in sugar or fast-digesting carbohydrates. What do you think your automatic response would be?

- Would this response help or hurt future progress?

- If you think this response might be detrimental to your continued success, what might be a more positive way of responding?

CONCLUSION

How to Maintain Your New, Addiction-Free Way of Eating

"Great works are performed, not by strength, but perseverance."

—DR. SAMUEL JOHNSON, ENGLISH AUTHOR

Many books will tell you the acceptable foods to eat and then send you off on your own to find out for yourself that the diets are not as easy to implement or maintain as they seem. Instead, we've designed this concluding chapter to give you some helpful hints, suggestions, and useful information that will aid you both as you adopt this new way of eating and as you maintain your new eating habits, after you have removed the majority of excess sugars and other carbohydrates from your diet and are living addiction-free.

A Look Back

The way of eating described in this book isn't revolutionary. Seventy years ago, when obesity and overeating were hardly a problem, almost everyone ate this way. Before the plethora of refined, processed foods and the addition of sugars to many foods, most people ate naturally and healthfully, consuming diets rich with meats, fish, cheese, vegetables, and sometimes fruit. Dessert was an occasional treat, not a daily occurrence. And as the Paleo Diet suggests,[1] even our ancestors ate primarily meats and fishes before they became hunter-gatherers or had begun farming. One of the arguments that the protein-rich Paleo Diet is more natural and fits our genetic makeup better than a high-sugar, high-carb diet is that our early ancestors had no sources of refined sugar or flour available.

The part of this book that *is* revolutionary is the concept that some foods, sugars, and other carbohydrates could be addictive. It might not have been a problem for our ancestors (both during the Paleolithic times and even as recently as seventy years ago) to eat a diet low in carbohydrates and added sugars, but in today's world, we have sweetened our diet and increased our portions so much that we are continually exposed to sugar-rich foods. We may now be dependent on these foods in a way that makes many of us unable to cut back on eating them, even when we know that we should.

Let's recap. In part one of this book, you learned about some reasons why your past diet attempts likely failed. You also learned some of the background information that you need to understand how much sugar you've really been eating. Next, you read about some of the criteria and processes that define and underlie addiction, and learned about recent research findings that suggest that certain foods, and sugar in particular, may be addictive if they are overconsumed.

Part two discussed a process that you can use to reduce your dependence on sugar and other carbohydrates by eliminating them or drastically reducing your intake of them. You also read about the types of foods you can eat on this plan, what foods to avoid, and what types of foods can serve as substitutes for the ones that you crave. You also learned about how to cope with withdrawal and cravings, which is a key component of breaking your addiction to sugars.

This information and your awareness of it is very important, but sometimes moving from awareness to action can be a challenge. How will you do it? How will you cut down on the foods that you have become so accustomed to eating? Some days this might seem like an impossible challenge, but if you have the proper tools and knowledge, you can do it.

Tips for Maintaining Your New Way of Eating

However, it isn't just certain types of food that you need to avoid. Often social situations and even certain individuals in your social circle can derail your eating plan, so this chapter will also address how to navigate these situations so that you can stay on track. And finally, this chapter will offer some concluding thoughts and more practical tips to help you implement this way of eating so that you can reduce your intake of (and as a result, your dependence on) sugar-rich foods.

TIP 1: APPLY WHAT YOU KNOW

As you've read this book, you've learned so many things that will help you to break the vicious cycle of addictive eating. You now understand why most diet plans fail, and how sugars and other carbohydrates can be addictive and lead many people to overeat them and cause unwanted weight gain. You also know about the places where sugars hide, and you have the information you need to make wise decisions with regard to selecting the right kinds of foods to eat. You know what situations and cues might promote overeating of addictive foods, and how to cope with them. You know how to deal with the physiological and psychological aspects of withdrawal from overuse of sugars, and how to assess and mitigate food cravings.

Now all you need is a few useful tips that will help you take all of that knowledge and put it into action. First, take notes; research suggests that active engagement in learning by taking notes benefits people's understanding and improves their performance on tests.[2] While there obviously won't be a written test after you read this book, your comprehension of the information discussed throughout will be crucial for your ability to pass the most important test of all—the test of whether you can finally break free of your dependence on unhealthy foods and implement a way of eating that will lead you to make wise food choices and achieve your goals.

This is one reason why the Food for Thought sections at the end of each chapter can be so helpful; not only do they ask you to reflect on aspects of your life (your eating patterns, your coping techniques, and so on), but they also ensure that you understand the concepts presented in each chapter so that you can apply them to *your* life. As you start to make grocery lists based on this information and lifestyle, you may want to write some of these phrases or facts on your list. This could serve as a friendly reminder as to why you are purchasing specific foods.

Next, turn your knowledge into action. For example, if you now know that you tend to snack on sugary cereal when you're watching television with your husband in the evening, apply the knowledge that you have regarding cues (for example: husband + television + relaxing on the couch = eating excess sugars) and change your environment. Watch television in a different room, or do something else to wind down. If you break the association, it will be easier for you to change this eating habit. It is important that you really think about your life and eating habits and, using the information in this book, make plans for how you can adjust your routine so you have an easier time giving up the foods that you know are bad for you.

Finally, you have to get in the habit of thinking ahead. This is very important, particularly at the beginning of the Sugar Freedom Plan, when you are starting to wean yourself off of sugar-rich drinks and foods. You know now that in many ways you are fighting an uphill battle: there will be a period of withdrawal, cravings, food cues, and stressors that cause you to want to throw in the towel. This is why it's important to plan out your meals and avoid situations in which you don't know how to react (for example, when someone asks you to eat a slice of birthday cake) or what to eat (for example, when you are invited to a friend's house for dinner).

TIP 2: TAKE CARE WHEN DINING OUT

Eating out with friends is a common part of our social lives. So, can you go to restaurants and still stay on track with your way of eating?

Yes, you can, but your challenge will be adjusting the foods you typically order. Be mindful of the fact that restaurants often have certain foods paired together, such as fish with french fries or potatoes. Remember that you can always ask for substitutions, such as steamed vegetables. So, whereas in the past you might have had a steak and a big baked potato, now you can still order your steak, and instead of the potato, have a big green salad with it, or a side of asparagus.

The bread basket—this is a big problem for some. If you're trying to reduce your carbohydrate intake, the last thing you need placed in front of you when you're hungry is a big basket of bread. You have two options: (1) Ask the people you're dining with if they want any bread, and if they say no, then tell the waiter not to bring bread. That way, you aren't wasting food, and you won't be tempted by it sitting in front of you while you wait for your meal. (2) If your party does want bread, then you'll have to use your willpower. Try asking for a beverage to be brought out right away so you have something to ingest while the others are noshing on bread. It helps if the people you are with know that you're trying to reduce your carbohydrate intake; they'll be less likely to ask you if you want some—and maybe they'll be less likely to want bread themselves.

Sometimes certain cuisines can be difficult to assess for their sugar and carbohydrate content. It's important to know the ingredients and contents of the foods that you are eating. Chinese food is tough; the reason it tastes good is because many of the dishes are chock-full of sugar. But there are seafood and stir-fry dishes in Chinese restaurants that fit beautifully with this diet, as long as you make some modifications to the items that are listed on the menu. For example, rice is a staple of most Asian dishes, so it's always difficult to eat them without a serving of carbohydrates. Remember, our modern food society is not designed around reducing your addiction to sugars and other carbohydrates, so you need to create your own food environment to suit your needs. Ask for the dishes without rice, and ask for the sauce on the side or left off completely. Do your homework: before you go to a restaurant, check online for the sugar and carbohydrate content of the foods. It also helps if you have a plan in mind before you get there as to what you want to order, so that you won't be caught off guard by the menu and feel pressed to order something before you think it through.

When it comes to fast-food restaurants, it's a bit more difficult. While you can eat on the run when needed, it's not a good idea to rely on this, as you tend to have fewer options and may be forced to eat something that you're trying to avoid. Even though places like McDonald's and Burger King have introduced salads to their menus that fit well into this diet, most of their lineup, even their breakfast lineup, is verboten. Also, remember that salad dressings often contain a lot of sugar, so be sure to check the label.

TIP 3: RESIST "FOOD PUSHERS"

We've all come face-to-face with food pushers at one time or another: your buddy asks you to get nachos and beer with him during half-time at a football game, your grandma shoves yet another one of her "world-famous" pastries at you after dinner, or your friend repeatedly offers you a piece of birthday cake. Despite our best efforts to maintain a balanced diet, these food pushers, with their encouraging words and persistence that "oh, you just have to try it" or "only one won't hurt" can lead you to unwise eating or drinking. So why do we often succumb to these pressures, and how can we stay on track in challenging social situations?

Let's take a closer look at a common situation that makes avoiding certain foods difficult: Your close friends have invited you to a barbeque at their house. When you arrive, there is a table full of appetizers—tortilla chips and salsa, pretzels, veggies and ranch dip.

The cooler beside it is full of various kinds of beer, soft drinks, and water. At the next table, there are platters full of hamburgers, hot dogs, and grilled chicken. Next to the platter is an array of condiments and accompaniments—ketchup, mayonnaise, cheese, lettuce, tomatoes, and onions. At the other end of the patio is the dessert table: cookies and fixings for ice-cream sundaes.

Yes, there are a lot of sugar-rich and unhealthy foods. No, you don't want to leave the party to avoid them. You are confident about applying what you know about food, and you approach the buffet. As you put some veggies on your plate, the hosts greet you and ask why you're not having some ranch dip with them. If you were at home, deviating from your healthy lifestyle wouldn't cross your mind. But there's something about being at a party and your friends' encouragement that leads you to waiver. Let's look at why.

According to the goal conflict model of eating, when dieters encounter a tasty food, they are faced with two conflicting goals: (1) enjoy the pleasure of eating or (2) weight control.[3] This model shows how the goal of eating can win over the goal of weight control. Why? Because we are surrounded by tasty foods, our mental representation of the weight control goal is inhibited.[4] Plus, the results of the weight control goal are long-term and may not be obvious at the moment, whereas the palatable food is right in front of us, so the result of the pleasurable eating goal will be immediate, however temporary. Because of these factors, we are more likely to focus on the goal of eating enjoyment. Tying this back to the party scenario, you're surrounded by foods and drinks you would not normally have at home, and your brain focuses on the pleasure of consuming them instead of your weight goals.

If we shift our focus to the social level, food environments and social relationships affect food choice.[5, 6, 7] Your food environment consists of the kinds of foods and ways of obtaining them that are available to you: grocery stores, fast-food chains, delis, ice-cream shops, convenience stores, and so on. Therefore, the foods made available to you will influence your choice of what to consume. In addition, scientists suggest that how well you know the individuals with whom you're eating can affect food intake. This means that the more comfortable you are around a person, the more relaxed you are, which facilitates consumption.[8, 9] Connecting this to the party situation suggests that your friendship with the hosts of the party makes you more relaxed and can lead you to loosen the restraint you planned on exercising.

Now that we have a better understanding of why certain people or situations can result in unwanted consumption of certain foods and drinks, let's think about some phrases you can use to help avoid the traps set by some situations and food pushers. To convey the firmness of your decision, it will be useful to use an assertive voice.

"You have to try some; I made it just for you"
"No thanks, I'm really not hungry."

"Since when are you picky about what you eat?"
"I've decided to focus on taking care of myself."

"Here, I got you another drink."
"No thanks, I have to drive tonight."

"A little piece won't hurt."
"My doctor says I shouldn't have any foods like that, so I'm going to follow what she recommended."

"You should have some. The hosts will be offended if you don't."
"I'll explain my decision to them. I know they will want me to be around for celebrations in the future, so it's best if I watch out for my own health now."

Another option is to simply tell people that you've decided to stop eating sugar. But anticipate some mixed reactions. Some people may be really interested and have a lot of questions about why you're doing it, what it is like, and how you do it. This can be your opportunity to teach people about what you have learned about addiction to food, hidden sugars, and ways to reduce or replace sugar in your diet.

However, some people may be more skeptical at first. Some may say things like "Well, if you aren't eating sugars, what the heck are you eating?" This is likely because when they reflect on their own diet, they see that it is loaded with sugars and carbohydrates, so cutting them out would not leave much else. Another typical reaction might be "I could never do that." Again, this can be an opportunity for you to pay it forward and to share what you have learned about cutting sugars from your diet and leading a happier, healthier lifestyle. You may turn a skeptic into a believer!

Another negative reaction that you may face is something like "That is dumb . . . you should just eat in moderation." People who respond in this way are probably not aware of the science behind sugar addiction and how moderation and self-control can be impossible if you're addicted to food. You can either (1) take this as an opportunity to tell them about the addictive nature of certain foods and how they can affect your brain and behavior or (2) shrug it off and change the topic.

Remember, you aren't obligated to explain yourself or your actions to anyone. It is your choice.

It's your body. You control what you consume. You are the only person who can decide which foods and drinks you will have. You know how to protect yourself against food pushers.

TIP 4: GET TO THE ROOT OF THE PROBLEM

Much of this book has focused on the nuts and bolts of addiction and how to conquer sugar addiction specifically, but a major point remains to be addressed that may be beneficial when trying to maintain a life that is free of sugar addiction. Just like food cravings may serve a certain function when we are stressed or upset, an addiction may serve a certain function for you as well, and it can be helpful to identify why this addiction began. Although you may be able to conquer your sugar or food addiction without a clear understanding of why the addiction developed, this understanding may be helpful going forward so that you know what signs to look for before falling back into a similar pattern.

There are multiple reasons that this addiction may have initially developed, including emotional, social, and even biochemical factors. Identifying when the addictive behaviors or even just overeating of sugary foods and drinks first began might provide clues as to what circumstances (internal or external) may have contributed to them. Again, the value of this is to be aware of when in particular you may be vulnerable to using these behaviors in the future so that you can be proactive.

Research reviewing narratives given by women addicted to alcohol or drugs found that drug use seemed to begin in an attempt to self-nurture.[10] The researchers point out, however, what most of us can surmise; that over the long run, this drug use resulted in negative consequences in various areas of their lives (work, family, and so on). This same process may take place with other types of addiction as well; maybe you used sugary foods or drinks to alleviate emotions that were difficult to sit with, but over time, has this behavior also caused problems in other aspects of your life? It may be helpful to contrast the reason(s) you started engaging in addictive behaviors regarding sugary foods and drinks with the effects these behaviors have caused over time. In fact, this group of researchers found that realizing that the costs were greater than the benefits of using alcohol or drugs was one of the key initial steps to the journey of recovery.

You may find that seeing a counselor or therapist is helpful when trying to understand why certain behaviors began and to identify healthy ways that these types of situations can be handled going forward. For instance, if you began overeating sugary foods as an escape from your emotions, a therapist may be able to help you identify and manage those emotions in a way that doesn't have you running to the pantry. In fact, this may be precisely why you turned to food in the first place—to avoid the difficulty of experiencing certain emotions, but consider again the cost-benefit analysis discussed above. In the moment, engaging in addictive behaviors may provide temporary relief, but it's just that—temporary—and the long-term consequences may be worse.

It is important to note, however, that an addiction to food may not necessarily be the result of an emotional reaction to something else in our life. Remember, our modern-day food environment is filled with things that can contribute to and perpetuate an addiction to food. In addition to constant cues and reminders of our favorite foods, we also tend to eat certain foods out of convenience. Also, as mentioned earlier, it is often less expensive to eat junk foods. Additionally, many of us may not have been taught good nutrition or eating habits. If you were raised drinking sugar-sweetened sodas and eating chips, these behaviors may seem normal and natural, and you may have a long history of overeating sugars without intention. Maybe you never gave much thought to the amount of sugar contained in many common foods. Maybe you just hate to cook! Whatever the reasons, it may be helpful to identify the factors that may have contributed to a pattern of overeating so that you are aware of what might influence you to overeat later on.

TIP 5: EAT BECAUSE YOU'RE HUNGRY,
NOT BECAUSE YOU'RE HAPPY

Continuing with this theme, research shows that people's emotions affect what, and when, they eat. We've offered a lot of information about why and what people eat for pleasure, but people also eat for other non-hunger-related reasons, such as stress[11] and even joy.[12] This probably doesn't come as a surprise, as many of us have, at one point or another, overeaten as a result of one or more of these feelings. But what can you do to control stress and other emotions?

Sleep! You might be overlooking the important impact of sleep on body weight. Research shows that people who get less sleep tend to weigh more.[13] Scientists have found that when people sleep less, motivation-related areas of the brain are highly activated at the sight of food,[14, 15] perhaps indicating that people who get less sleep may be more inclined to overeat. Biologically, this makes sense too, as there are links between lack of sleep and dysfunction of satiety signals.[16] With high-stress, fast-paced lifestyles, people may sacrifice sleep in an attempt to make more time for work or spending time with others—things that add to people's quality of life and make them happy. However, forgoing sleep can have a negative effect on body weight, so while you may be happy to have time for some things that give you joy, you may be sacrificing your health.

What about when you are awake? What can you do to take command and control of your emotions while you're up and about throughout your day? A growing body of literature supports the benefits of mindfulness of food choice.[17, 18, 19] Mindfulness involves taking the time to consider factors such as why you are eating, how you are feeling, and what you are accomplishing for yourself by consuming a given food; based on this thought process, a person makes a thoughtful decision about whether or not to eat, what to eat, or how much to eat. For some people, yoga and meditation are methods of incorporating this type of thinking into their lives. However, other people may prefer different forms of self-reflection. These may include writing or typing your thoughts and emotions in a journal, on a notepad, or on a computerized document, stating your thoughts and feelings aloud before acting, or keeping a notepad on your refrigerator or pantry so that you can note how you're feeling before eating.

TIP 6: SET SHORT-TERM AND LONG-TERM GOALS

Before you begin a diet plan, or any new plan at all, you need goals. However, some people set goals that require drastic change in a short amount of time, or that don't take into account their lifestyle and current set of circumstances. This section will outline how to set practical and realistic goals over time.

Goal setting is a strategy used across a variety of disciplines, from athletes to physicians and their patients, to help people succeed. Goals provide reference points for progress and are useful for self-discipline and self-regulation. There is a plethora of smart phone apps, books, and websites that incorporate goal setting, each with its own special features and organization schemes. There are many options for developing and keeping track of goals, so let's start with some of the basics involved in goal setting.

KNOW YOURSELF. First and foremost, consider your personality traits. What motivates you? How do you like to tackle new situations—alone, in a group, with a friend, or with a combination of these? How do you respond to stress? How do you hold yourself accountable for your actions? Taking an honest look at yourself and writing down information about your strengths, weaknesses, habits, and lifestyle will enable you to design personalized and realistic goals. After answering these questions, answer these two as well: Why do you want to change your lifestyle? How do you define success in regard to this diet plan?

THINK ABOUT THE PAST. Most people agree that to know where you're going, it's helpful to know where you came from. What has led you to succeed? What has made becoming successful a struggle? How have you dealt with adversity or challenges in the past? By examining and learning from previous events and experiences, you can apply this knowledge as you look to the future.

USE POSITIVE PHRASING. A vital aspect of attaining your goals lies in how you phrase them. Try to use specific and concise language. This will help you clearly define your goals and remember them easily. For example, let's say you want to lose ten pounds. An effective way of phrasing this goal would be "I will lose ten pounds in eighteen weeks." In doing so, you have set a time frame that gives you some flexibility to adjust to your changes in lifestyle, you've only used a few words, and you've used positive, determined language that suggests that you believe in your ability to achieve this goal within the given time frame by saying "I will lose" instead of "I hope to lose" or "I would like to lose."

MAKE YOUR GOALS SHORT-TERM. Select two elements from this book and turn them into short-term goals. For example: "This week, I will not drink sugar-filled soda." Make sure to include a small time frame and to set a goal that involves a small change. At the end of the allotted amount of time, check in with yourself to see if you were successful in achieving your goal. If you were successful, congratulations! Now set another short-term goal, and keep setting them until you reach your long-term goal (see below). If you didn't reach your short-term goal within the allotted time frame, spend some time evaluating where you went wrong and use this information to help you achieve the next short-term goal you set.

LOOK TO THE LONG TERM. You have set a series of short-term goals, and now you can to look at long-term goals. Once you have decided on a goal, try to set a realistic time frame. The time frame is entirely of your choosing—one month, three months, one year, five years. This goal might sound something like "In six months, I will lose X pounds." As you know, you define success, so your goals can reflect what you want. Be confident because you have the knowledge it takes to set realistic and informed goals.

TIP 7: BE CONSISTENT

The idea that these modifications in your diet are meant to result in a lifestyle change has been mentioned many times throughout the book. This means that you can apply what you have learned about the neuroscience and psychology behind eating today, tomorrow, and for years to come. It persists across birthday celebrations, dinner parties, and holidays.

All of this change will likely take some time. You may need to adjust to eating different foods, increasing the amount of hours you sleep, or thinking before eating. You may end up tweaking some of your goals to make them more realistic as you find what works for you. All of this is fine! Use this knowledge in ways that work best for you.

The key is to be consistent. There is evidence that people who maintain their diet throughout the week are more likely to maintain their weight loss over the following year than people who diet more strictly on weekdays.[20] Upholding consistent behaviors helps to serve as a baseline; that means that you can easily identify when you deviate from your normal behavior so that you can make a change to get back in the direction you want to go. By consistently focusing on your goals, you can achieve them in the face of slipups, food pushers, and any curveballs that life throws at you.

The Final Word: Eating and Living without Your Addiction

As mentioned in the introduction, this is much more than a diet book. It involves much greater change in your life than just a way to lose weight would. If this book were *only* about losing weight, it would still be a good thing because excess weight may contribute to several health problems and can wreak havoc on self-esteem and confidence. But this book offers much more: it really presents a new way of living. It may sound hokey, but the results can be that dramatic.

These pages suggest changes to your diet that really can have a meaningful impact on how you feel and live. You'll have more energy, and you'll feel better after adopting this plan. You'll have fewer mood swings as you will have normalized your blood sugar and insulin levels, instead of living through constant surges and dips brought on by overeating sugars. You'll probably also feel less anxious and depressed when you are no longer suffering mini withdrawals between your dosages of sugar.

Maybe the best part of this diet plan is that you will no longer feel guilty. Guilt is the addict's worst friend. Addiction has the ability to alter our thinking processes. And it can impair our rational thinking in the short run, but even addicts have periods of self-reflection when they realize their lives are not going in the direction they want them to. They may blame their addiction, but this doesn't minimize the guilt they feel. People who are addicted sometimes feel enormous guilt because they feel they should be able to control their own actions and behavior. This guilt can prevent people from gaining the self-confidence and inner strength needed to really conquer addictions. Guilt can be self-defeating. Guilt can keep you down.

There will certainly be skeptics, and some may say things like "What fun could there be in life if you get rid of sugary foods?" So is this a boring life? Let's look. Your old addictive life may have been full of processed foods, stress, and wasting a great deal of time on nonproductive behaviors revolving around food. What about your new life? Now you'll be eating healthy. You'll be more active and more energized. You'll be happier with the way you look and feel, and this will rub off on to how you interact with others. Once you regain your ability to decide your life plans and goals for yourself and pursue them without the damaging influence of your addiction interfering, life is definitely not boring. In fact, there is a whole new world out there to be discovered once you kick your addiction.

To emphasize how dramatically your life will change on this diet plan, let's take a minute and describe what a typical day in your life might look like before and after you adopt this diet.

Your typical day before adopting this way of eating might read like this: Your alarm blasts in the morning and you hit the snooze button at least twice so you can sleep an additional ten or fifteen minutes. You finally wake, but you feel terrible. You have no energy, and you don't feel like getting out of bed. Your whole body aches. You eventually pull yourself out of bed and run downstairs to put on coffee and eat some Cap'n Crunch cereal that you bought for your kids. On weekends (when you aren't facing your usual morning rush), you might treat yourself to pancakes, waffles, or French toast with lots of syrup, but after eating it, you feel even sleepier and wish you could just head back up to bed for a midmorning nap.

Later, you eat some M&Ms and wash them down with a cup of coffee, but you don't feel any better. You go out to lunch and eat an entire plate of spaghetti or lasagna and wonder if you can fit under your desk for an afternoon nap. You come back to the office, but you don't feel like working. So you do a mediocre job with the assignments you are given. Then you feel guilty because you realize you didn't give it your best. You head home as soon as you can, whip up a quick meal (maybe tonight is macaroni and cheese night, again), and retreat to your television. You retire to your bed but never seem to be able to get a good night's rest (perhaps because you are wired from all of the sugar you have been eating).

Now, let's contrast this with your new life after having adopted this diet. You won't believe this, but now you might even wake up *before* your alarm. You've left the shades up in the bedroom and as soon as the sun comes up, your eyes open. But instead of feeling lousy and wishing you could sleep more, you literally pop out of bed and feel like a million bucks. You don't know what to do first. You can't wait to feel that wonderful shower on your face and back, but you also know that if you exercise each morning, you will feel better throughout the day. Exercising is no longer a prison sentence; you are not chained to a treadmill. Now you get to go out and enjoy nature, the fresh air, and the natural beauty. Because you've gotten out of bed so early, after you work out, you have plenty of time to cook a good breakfast and eat it at a leisurely pace without worrying about being late for work. You cook up an egg omelet with sausage, cheese, and mushrooms and wash it down with a tall drink of water.

You get to work on time and you feel great, and it's reflected in your productivity. Sure, your coworkers still have their funny personality quirks that used to drive you crazy, but now for some reason they no longer bother you as much. For lunch, you go out with the girls in marketing and find a restaurant that serves you a beautiful piece of fish with butter and almonds on it with a small side order of broccoli, cauliflower, and carrots.

You have a snack in the afternoon, not of raisins or dried fruits glued together with sugar and honey in the form of a bar, but instead a small bag of almonds and cashews. You come home and decide to have your favorite meal, barbecued spareribs with sugar-free barbecue sauce. There's a side dish of green beans with butter and pepper, and you top it off with a beautiful slice of melon for dessert. After dinner, you don't want to flop in front of the television because you still have lots of energy; instead, you decide to do some of those things that you've been wanting to do in your spare time.

You probably think this is an exaggeration, but this is what testimonials from people who have changed their way of eating and broken free from their addiction to sugars and other carbohydrates convey. Try it for yourself—why not? What do you have to lose, besides weight and an addiction?

APPENDIX: SUGAR EQUIVALENCY TABLE

Sugar equivalence is a concept that John first came up with to capture how much sugar and fast-digesting carbohydrates are in a food as a percent of its total weight. You can see from our table that foods vary enormously in their sugar equivalency.

The Sugar Equivalency Table was compiled using data provided by the USDA, which lists nutrition facts for thousands of foods. The simple formula used to create the values you see in the table takes a 100-gram sample of food, measures how many grams of sugar are in that 100-gram sample, and adds 75 percent of the nonfiber, nonsugar carbohydrate grams to account for the fact that starches, like sugar, can also cause an increase in glucose levels and thus insulin levels (to break down the glucose).

A general rule of thumb to use when reading the Sugar Equivalency Table is that the lower the sugar equivalency in a food, the better it fits this way of eating. For example, most meats and poultry have sugar equivalency values of 0 because they have no sugar and no carbohydrates in them, but candies and cakes have sugar equivalency numbers in the 50 to 70 range, and so are to be avoided on this plan. As a general guideline, foods under 5 are acceptable on the diet, foods scoring between 5 and 10 can be consumed but their quantity should be monitored, and anything over 10 should be fairly restricted or avoided. The food items in the table are sorted generally by type of food.

It's not enough to say that you shouldn't consume foods with high sugar equivalency. You also have to be mindful of the amount or weight of the food that you're consuming. We are all human, and at times, we might give into our impulses to eat foods that we're trying to avoid. If you regress one night and have a small plate of spaghetti, all is not lost; cooked macaroni has a sugar equivalency of only 14. It could be worse. It's important to note, however, that the size of your portions does matter. It's not a good idea to have a one-third portion of pasta whenever you want because of thinking that a one-third portion falls within the "safe range" in terms of sugar equivalency. The Sugar Equivalency Table isn't designed to work like that.

If you consume low-sugar-equivalency foods like meats, vegetables, poultry, and seafood, you'll lessen your dependence on sugars. As a result, you'll stop eating because you crave sugars and instead begin to eat based on true hunger, rational decision making, and occasionally pleasure. Your food choices will no longer be driven by the "need" or compulsion to consume certain foods, which may stem from an addiction. You'll also find that you can consume as much sugar- or carb-free food as you like because you will only *want* to eat as much as you need to satisfy your hunger, not your addiction. The beauty of this approach is that it reduces complex nutritional information about individual foods down to one simple number. It's not an exact science, but for people who are trying to monitor their sugar intake and lose weight, it can be extremely helpful. Can you imagine picking up each food item in a grocery store, looking at its nutrition label, and trying to do this calculation in order to arrive at an estimate of how much sugar and nonfibrous, nonsugar carbohydrates are contained in the food as a percentage of total weight? No way. It would be next to impossible. You shouldn't need a calculator to go to the grocery store. So instead, all you need to do is refer to a table that summarizes all of that information into one number.

As this table demonstrates, you don't need to memorize the sugar equivalency of every single food item in the world to be successful on this diet as long as you primarily consume food items that belong to groups of foods that have low sugar equivalencies and stay away from those that have high sugar equivalencies. There are some food groups, like fruits and vegetables, that are in the mid-range of sugar equivalency, but some may need to be examined more closely using the Sugar Equivalency Table.

Until you feel comfortable that you have a good idea of the relative sugar equivalency levels associated with these different food groups, you might want to copy down some of the items on this list and stick it in your wallet or purse. It can serve as a helpful reminder when you're in the grocery store or out to eat at a restaurant.

SUGAR EQUIVALENCY TABLE

The following table provides a single number, or "sugar equivalence," for common food and drink items. Sugar equivalency values do *not* take into account other factors that are also important when making food choices, such as the number of vitamins a food or drink offers. This table is meant as a guide to help you assess the relative sugar content in many popular foods, which may be useful when thinking about which foods to avoid.

FOOD ITEM	TOTAL SUGAR EQUIVALENCY
BEVERAGES	
Apple juice from frozen concentrate, unsweetened	11
Club soda	0
Coffee, brewed, espresso, decaffeinated	0
Coffee, brewed from grounds	0
Coffee, instant	0

FOOD ITEM	TOTAL SUGAR EQUIVALENCY
Energy drink, Monster	11
Energy drink, Powerade, lemon-lime flavor	7
Energy drink, Powerade zero Ion4, calorie-free, assorted flavors	0
Energy drink, Rockstar	13
Fruit punch drink, canned	12
Gatorade, fruit-flavored, ready to drink	6

FOOD ITEM	TOTAL SUGAR EQUIVALENCY
BEVERAGES, continued	
Grape drink, canned	15
Grape juice, unsweetened	14
Lemonade from powdered mix	4
Lemonade, low-calorie, from powdered mix w/aspartame	1
Orange juice, raw	10
Soda, cola or Dr. Pepper type, low-calorie w/caffeine and sodium saccharin	0
Soda, cola w/caffeine	9
Soda, cola w/o caffeine	11
Soda, cream	13
Soda, ginger ale	9
Soda, grape	8
Soda, lemon-lime w/caffeine	10
Soda, orange	9
Soymilk, original and vanilla, unfortified	5
Tea, black	0
Tea, chamomile, brewed	0
Tea, instant, sweetened with sugar, lemon-flavored, from powdered mix	8
Tea, instant, sweetened with saccharin, lemon-flavored, from powdered mix	0
Tea, instant, unsweetened, from powdered mix	0
V8 organic vegetable juice	4
Water, bottled, Perrier	0
Wine, nonalcoholic	1
BREADS, CAKES, AND COOKIES	
Bagels, cinnamon-raisin	41
Bagels, oat bran	38
Bagels, plain (includes onion, poppy, sesame)	42
Biscuits, plain or buttermilk, frozen, baked	36
Bread, banana, prepared from recipe, made w/margarine	40
Bread, cornbread, dry mix, prepared	34
Bread, egg	35
Bread, French or vienna (includes sourdough)	41
Bread, Italian	36
Bread, oat bran	28
Bread, oatmeal	35
Bread, pumpernickel	31
Bread, raisin, enriched	37
Bread, reduced-calorie, oat bran	23
Bread, rye	33
Bread, wheat	35
Bread, wheat bran	35
Bread, wheat germ	36
Bread, white, and soft bread crumbs	36
Bread, whole-wheat	27
Bread crumbs, dry, plain	52
Bread sticks, plain	49
Bread stuffing, dry mix, prepared	15
Brownies	56
Cake, angel food	42
Cake, Boston cream	40
Cake, cheesecake	24
Cake, chocolate w/chocolate frosting	48
Cake, cinnamon coffeecake w/crumb topping	34
Cake, coffeecake, cheese	32
Cake, pineapple upside-down	37
Cake, pound, prepared w/butter	36
Cake, shortcake, biscuit-type	36
Cake, snack, creme-filled, chocolate w/ frosting	52
Cake, snack, creme-filled, sponge	57
Cake, sponge	55
Cake, white w/coconut frosting	61
Cake, white w/o frosting	51
Cake, yellow w/chocolate frosting	51
Cookies, animal crackers	58
Cookies, Archway home-style oatmeal	58
Cookies, Archway home-style reduced-fat ginger snaps	65

FOOD ITEM	TOTAL SUGAR EQUIVALENCY
Cookies, Archway home-style sugar-free oatmeal	49
Cookies, chocolate-chip, higher-fat	55
Cookies, fig bars	61
Cookies, graham crackers, plain or honey	63
Cookies, oatmeal	56
Cookies, oatmeal, special dietary	58
Cookies, oatmeal, w/o raisins	50
Cookies, peanut butter	51
Cookies, peanut butter sandwich, special dietary	38
Cookies, sugar	60
Cookies, vanilla wafers, higher-fat	52
Cookies, vanilla wafers, lower-fat	63
Crackers, cheese	44
Crackers, melba toast	53
Crackers, Nabisco graham	60
Crackers, standard snack-type	46
Crackers, wheat	51
Croissants, butter	35
Doughnuts, cake-type, plain, chocolate-coated or frosted	44
Doughnuts, cake-type, plain (includes unsugared, old-fashioned)	37
Doughnuts, yeast-leavened, glazed, (includes honey buns)	41
English muffin, plain (includes sourdough)	31
French toast, made w/2% milk	19
Hush puppies	33
Ice cream cones, cake or wafer-type	59
Muffins, blueberry	43
Muffins, corn	38
Muffins, oat bran	35
Muffins, plain, made w/2% milk	29
Muffins, wheat bran, toaster-type w/raisins	37
Pancakes, buttermilk	22
Pancakes, Eggo buttermilk	30
Pancakes, plain	21

FOOD ITEM	TOTAL SUGAR EQUIVALENCY
Pastry, cinnamon Danish	37
Pastry, sweet rolls, cheese	32
Pastry, sweet rolls, cinnamon w/raisins	44
Pie, apple	28
Pie, banana cream	27
Pie, cherry	33
Pie, chocolate cream	24
Pie, coconut cream, prepared from mix, no-bake type	21
Pie, lemon meringue	40
Pie, peach	26
Pie, pecan	49
Pie, pumpkin	29
Pie crust, graham cracker	57
Pie crust, standard-type, prepared from dry mix	39
Pop-Tarts, Kellogg's apple-cinnamon	62
Pop-Tarts, Kellogg's brown sugar cinnamon	54
Pop-Tarts, Kellogg's strawberry	61
Rolls, dinner, egg	37
Rolls, dinner, plain	39
Rolls, dinner, whole wheat	35
Rolls, hamburger or hotdog, plain	38
Taco shells, baked	44
Waffles, Eggo low-fat nutri-grain	29
Waffles, plain	25
CANDIES, SNACKS, AND SWEETS	
Candies, butterscotch	88
Candies, caramels	74
Candies, fudge, vanilla	82
Candies, gumdrops	89
Candies, hard	89
Candies, M&M's milk chocolate	67
Candies, M&M's peanut	55
Candies, milk chocolate–coated peanuts	43
Candies, milk chocolate–coated raisins	65

FOOD ITEM	TOTAL SUGAR EQUIVALENCY
CANDIES, SNACKS, AND SWEETS, continued	
Candies, milk chocolate w/almonds	46
Candies, Nestle Bit-o'-Honey	72
Candies, peanut brittle	64
Candies, Raisinets chocolate-covered raisins	66
Candies, Reese's Pieces	56
Candies, Rolo caramels in milk chocolate	66
Candies, Starburst fruit chews	76
Candies, Tootsie roll, chocolate flavor	80
Candies, Twizzlers nibs cherry bits	72
Candies, York peppermint patties	75
Candy bar, 100 Grand	65
Candy bar, 3 Musketeers	74
Candy bar, Almond Joy	53
Candy bar, Baby Ruth	61
Candy bar, Kit Kat	60
Candy bar, Mars, almond	59
Candy bar, Milky Way	68
Candy bar, Mounds	53
Candy bar, Mr. Goodbar	50
Candy bar, Skor toffee	60
Candy bar, Snickers	57
Candy bar, Twix caramel cookie	60
Chips, bagel, plain	48
Chips, banana	47
Chips, potato, barbecue flavor	38
Chips, potato fat-free, salted	58
Chips, potato, sour cream and onion flavor	35
Chips, tortilla, yellow plain	47
Chocolate, baking, unsweetened, squares	10
Chocolate, milk	55
Chocolate, semisweet	57
Chocolate, white	59
Cornnuts, nacho flavor	48
Egg custard, baked	11

FOOD ITEM	TOTAL SUGAR EQUIVALENCY
Frosting, chocolate, creamy	61
Frosting, vanilla, creamy	67
Gelatin powder, unsweetened	0
Granola bars, chewy, reduced-sugar	55
Granola bars, hard, chocolate chip	51
Granola bars, hard, peanut	53
Granola bars, hard, plain	51
Granola bars, Quaker oatmeal to go, all flavors	61
Granola bars, soft, uncoated, plain	47
Granola bars, soft, w/milk chocolate coating, chocolate chip	45
Honey	82
Ice cream, Breyers, 98% fat-free vanilla	24
Ice cream, Breyers, lite vanilla	25
Ice cream, Breyers, no sugar added, vanilla	18
Ice cream cone, chocolate-covered, w/nuts, flavors other than chocoloate	31
Ice cream, fat-free fudgesicle bars	24
Ice cream, fat-free, no sugar added, flavors other than chocolate	18
Ice cream sandwich	32
Ice cream, soft serve, chocolate	21
Ice cream, vanilla, rich	22
Ice pops, sugar-free, orange, cherry, or grape popsicles	4
Jams and preserves	63
Jellies	65
Marmalade, orange	64
Meal-replacement bar, Clif bar	51
Meal-replacement bar, Power bar, chocolate	55
Meal-replacement bar, Slim-fast, milk chocolate peanut	48
Molasses	70
Popcorn, air-popped	48
Popcorn, caramel-coated, w/peanuts	69
Popcorn, oil-popped	28

FOOD ITEM	TOTAL SUGAR EQUIVALENCY
Pork skins, plain	0
Pretzels, hard, plain, salted	58
Pretzels, soft, unsalted	52
Pudding, chocolate	22
Pudding, rice	17
Pudding, tapioca, fat-free	20
Pudding, tapioca, prepared w/whole milk	15
Pudding, vanilla	21
Pudding, vanilla, fat-free	19
Sugar, brown	98
Sugar, granulated	100
Sugar, powdered	99
Syrups, chocolate	59
Syrups, corn, lite	64
Syrups, Hershey's genuine chocolate flavor lite	33
Syrups, table blends, pancake	51
Syrups, table blends, pancake, reduced-calorie	42
Toppings, butterscotch or caramel	49
Toppings, marshmallow cream	71
Toppings, pineapple	55
Trail mix, Nature Valley granola bars chewy	62
Trail mix, regular	34
Trail mix, tropical	49

CANNED AND FROZEN FOOD

FOOD ITEM	TOTAL SUGAR EQUIVALENCY
Beef barley soup, Campbell's chunky, healthy request	5
Beef stew, Campbell's chunky	6
Beef stroganoff soup, Campbell's chunky	5
Chicken noodle soup, reduced-sodium, canned	2
Frozen, corn dogs	24
Frozen, Hot Pockets chicken, broccoli, and cheddar croissant sandwich	24
Frozen, Lasagna, cheese	10
Frozen, Lasagna w/meat and sauce	9

FOOD ITEM	TOTAL SUGAR EQUIVALENCY
Frozen, Lean Pockets, ham and cheddar	25
Frozen, pot pie, beef	16
Frozen, pot pie, turkey	12
Frozen, rice bowl w/chicken	17
Macaroni and cheese, canned	8
Ravioli, cheese-filled, canned	10
Ravioli, meat-filled, w/tomato sauce or meat sauce, canned	10
Spaghettios, original	11
Tortellini w/cheese filling	34

CEREALS

FOOD ITEM	TOTAL SUGAR EQUIVALENCY
All-Bran complete wheat flakes, Kellogg's	50
All-Bran original, Kellogg's	38
Apple Jacks, Kellogg's	70
Cap'n Crunch	73
Cheerios	49
Cocoa Puffs	68
Corn Chex	60
Corn Flakes, Kellogg's	66
Corn grits	11
Cracklin' Oat Bran	52
Cream of Rice	8
Cream of Wheat	8
Cocoa Krispies, Kellogg's	73
Granola w/fruit, low-fat, Nature Valley	65
Granola w/raisins, low-fat, Kellogg's	61
Grape-Nuts	57
Honey Nut Cheerios	62
Honey Nut Shredded Wheat	60
Honey Smacks, Kellogg's	78
Lucky Charms	66
Oatmeal	8
Oatmeal, instant	17
Raisin Bran, Kellogg's	57
Wheat germ	28

FOOD ITEM	TOTAL SUGAR EQUIVALENCY
DAIRY AND EGG PRODUCTS	
Cheese, American	6
Cheese, blue	2
Cheese, Brie	0
Cheese, Camembert	0
Cheese, Cheddar	1
Cheese, cottage, creamed	3
Cheese, cottage, 1% fat	3
Cheese, cream	4
Cheese, feta	4
Cheese, Gouda	2
Cheese, Gruyère	0
Cheese, mozzarella, whole milk	2
Cheese, Muenster	1
Cheese, Parmesan, grated	3
Cheese, provolone	2
Cheese, Swiss	4
Cheese product, Kraft American nonfat process	10
Cheese spread, Kraft Velveeta process	9
Cream, sour, cultured	3
Cream, sour, fat-free	12
Cream, sour, reduced-fat	5
Cream, whipped, pressurized	11
Egg, white	1
Egg, whole	1
Egg, yolk	3
Eggnog	8
Milk, 2% fat	5
Milk, chocolate, whole-milk	10
Milk, fat-free or skim	5
Milk shake, thick chocolate	21
Milk shake, thick vanilla	18
Milk, whole, 3.25% fat	5
Yogurt, fruit, low-fat, 9 g protein per 8 oz.	19
Yogurt, plain, low-fat, 12 g protein per 8 oz.	7
Yogurt, plain, whole-milk, 8 g protein per 8 oz.	5

FOOD ITEM	TOTAL SUGAR EQUIVALENCY
FAST FOOD AND RESTAURANT FOOD	
Applebee's double-crunch shrimp	17
Biscuit, w/egg and bacon	14
Burger King cheeseburger	17
Burger King croissant sandwich w/sausage, egg, and cheese	13
Burger King french fries	28
Burger King french toast sticks	32
Burger King hamburger, double whopper w/cheese	10
Burger King hamburger, whopper w/cheese	13
Burger King hash brown rounds	24
Burrito, w/beans	25
Cheeseburger, single	23
Chili con carne w/beans, canned	8
Chinese restaurant, beef and vegetables	5
Chinese restaurant, chicken chow mein	6
Chinese restaurant, egg drop soup	3
Chinese restaurant, egg rolls	19
Chinese restaurant, fried rice	23
Chinese restaurant, General Tso's chicken	20
Chinese restaurant, hot and sour soup	3
Chinese restaurant, kung pao chicken	5
Chinese, restaurant, lemon chicken	16
Chinese restaurant, shrimp and vegetables	3
Chinese restaurant, sweet-and-sour chicken	20
Chinese restaurant, sweet-and-sour pork	19
Chinese restaurant, wonton soup	4
Cracker Barrel, chicken tenderloin platter, fried, from kid's menu	13
Cracker Barrel, grilled sirloin steak	0
Denny's, fried shrimp	14
Denny's, top sirloin steak	0
Domino's cheese pizza, classic hand-tossed crust	24
Domino's pepperoni pizza, ultimate deep-dish crust	23

FOOD ITEM	TOTAL SUGAR EQUIVALENCY
Hamburger, single	26
Hotdog, plain	14
Kentucky Fried Chicken fried chicken, extra-crispy, w/skin and breading	16
Kentucky Fried Chicken fried chicken, original recipe, breast-meat	0
Kentucky Fried Chicken fried chicken, original recipe, w/skin and breading	13
Kentucky Fried Chicken popcorn chicken	15
Kentucky Fried Chicken potato wedges	23
Latino, rice pudding	22
Latino, tamale, corn	19
Little Caesars original cheese pizza, regular crust	23
McDonald's big mac	15
McDonald's chicken nuggets	12
McDonald's chicken sandwich, classic, premium crispy	19
McDonald's chicken sandwich, classic, premium grilled	17
McDonald's egg muffin	15
McDonald's filet of fish	21
McDonald's french fries	26
McDonald's hamburger	24
McDonald's hamburger, quarter pounder	17
McDonald's hamburger, quarter pounder w/cheese	15
McDonald's hot fudge sundae	29
McDonald's hotcakes and sausage	33
McDonald's salad, bacon ranch w/grilled chicken	2
McDonald's salad, caesar w/grilled chicken	2
McDonald's salad, fruit and walnut	16
McDonald's salad, side	3
McDonald's sausage biscuit	20
McDonald's vanilla triple-thick shake	25
Nachos, w/cheese	24
Papa John's cheese pizza, original crust	24
Pizza Hut cheese pizza, hand-tossed crust	24

FOOD ITEM	TOTAL SUGAR EQUIVALENCY
Pizza Hut cheese pizza, pan crust	22
Pizza Hut pepperoni pizza, hand-tossed crust	23
Popeyes biscuit	30
Popeyes fried chicken, mild, w/skin and breading	17
Popeyes spicy chicken strips	13
Potato salad w/egg	12
Pulled pork in barbecue sauce	17
Submarine sandwich, w/cold cuts	17
Sundae, hot fudge	23
Taco Bell bean burrito	21
Taco Bell burrito supreme w/beef	13
Taco Bell nachos	24
Taco Bell original taco w/beef, cheese, and lettuce	12
Taco salad	9
T.G.I. Friday's chicken fingers, from kid's menu	8
T.G.I. Friday's fried mozzarella	17
T.G.I. Friday's shrimp, breaded	9
Wendy's chicken fillet sandwich, home-style	15
Wendy's chicken nuggets	11
Wendy's frosty dairy dessert	15
Wendy's hamburger, classic single w/cheese	10

FATS, OILS, DRESSINGS, AND SAUCES

FOOD ITEM	TOTAL SUGAR EQUIVALENCY
Butter, salted	0
Butter, unsalted	0
Fat, chicken	0
Fat, turkey	0
Horseradish, prepared	8
Margarine-butter blend, soybean oil and butter	1
Margarine, stick, 80% fat, w/salt	1
Oil, coconut	0
Oil, cod liver	0
Oil, corn	0

FOOD ITEM	TOTAL SUGAR EQUIVALENCY
FATS, OILS, DRESSINGS, AND SAUCES, continued	
Oil, olive	0
Oil, palm	0
Oil, peanut	0
Oil, rice bran	0
Oil, sesame	0
Oil, soybean	0
Oil, soybean, partially hydrogenated	0
Oil, sunflower, linoleic (less than 60%)	0
Oil, wheat germ	0
Salad dressing, 1000 island	15
Salad dressing, 1000 island, reduced-fat	21
Salad dressing, blue or Roquefort	4
Salad dressing, French	16
Salad dressing, French, reduced-fat	27
Salad dressing, French, w/o salt	16
Salad dressing, Italian	10
Salad dressing, Italian, reduced-fat	5
Salad dressing, Italian, w/o salt	10
Salad dressing, Kraft miracle whip free, nonfat	13
Salad dressing, Russian	28
Salad dressing, Russian, low-calorie	26
Sauce, cocktail	23
Sauce, steak, tomato-based	18
Sauce, sweet-and-sour	33
Sauce, tartar	11
Shortening, lard and vegetable oil	0
Shortening, partially hydrogenated soybean-cottonseed	0
Vegetable oil, butter tub, w/salt	1
Vegetable oil spread, fat-free, tub	3
Vinegar, balsamic	17
Vinegar, distilled	0
Vinegar, red wine	0

FOOD ITEM	TOTAL SUGAR EQUIVALENCY
FRUITS	
Apples, dehydrated, sulfured, uncooked	81
Apples, dried, sulfured, uncooked	57
Apples, raw, with skin	11
Applesauce, canned, sweetened	16
Apricots, dehydrated, sulfured, uncooked	62
Apricots, dried, sulfured, uncooked	55
Apricots, raw	9
Avocados, raw	2
Bananas, dehydrated, or banana powder	71
Bananas, raw	18
Blackberries, raw	5
Blueberries, raw	12
Cantaloupe, raw	8
Cherries, sour, red, raw	10
Cherries, sweet, raw	14
Cranberries, raw	7
Figs, dried, uncooked	53
Figs, raw	16
Fruit cocktail, canned in heavy syrup w/liquid	18
Grapefruit, raw	7
Grapes, red or green, raw	17
Honeydew melon, raw	8
Kiwifruit, raw	11
Lemon juice, raw	6
Lemons, raw, without peel	6
Limes, raw	6
Mangos, raw	14
Olives, ripe, canned	2
Oranges, raw	9
Papayas, raw	9
Peaches, raw	8
Pears, raw	12
Pineapple, raw	11
Plantains, raw	26

FOOD ITEM	TOTAL SUGAR EQUIVALENCY
Plums, dried prunes, uncooked	52
Plums, raw	10
Prunes, dehydrated (low-moisture), uncooked	67
Raisins, seedless	71
Raspberries, raw	5
Rhubarb, raw	2
Strawberries, raw	5
Tangerines (mandarin oranges), raw	11
GRAINS AND PASTAS	
Barley, hulled	42
Buckwheat	46
Corn, yellow	50
Cornmeal, whole-grain, yellow	52
Cornstarch	68
Macaroni, cooked	22
Noodles, Chinese, chow mein	40
Noodles, egg, cooked	18
Noodles, rice, cooked	18
Oat bran, cooked	7
Pasta, fresh, cooked	19
Rice, brown, long-grain, cooked	16
Rice, white, long-grain, cooked	21
Rice, white, short-grain, cooked	22
Spaghetti, cooked	22
Wheat flour, white, 9% protein	58
MEATS AND POULTRY	
Bacon	0
Beef franks, Oscar Mayer weiners	2
Beef, ground	0
Beef ribs	0
Bologna, beef	3
Bologna, beef, Oscar Mayer	2
Bratwurst, pork and beef, link	3
Chicken, broilers or fryers, breast, meat, and skin, raw	0

FOOD ITEM	TOTAL SUGAR EQUIVALENCY
Chicken, broilers or fryers, meat and skin, battered and fried	7
Chicken, broilers or fryers, meat and skin, raw	0
Chicken, broilers or fryers, meat only, raw	0
Chicken, broilers or fryers, meat, skin, giblets, and neck, raw	0
Chicken, cornish game hens, meat and skin, raw	0
Chicken nuggets, frozen, cooked	9
Duck breast, meat and skin, roasted	0
Duck, domesticated, meat and skin, raw	0
Frankfurter, beef and pork	1
Frankfurter, turkey	3
Goose, domesticated, meat and skin, raw	0
Ham, sliced, prepackaged, 96% fat-free	1
Knockwurst, pork and beef	2
Lamb, domestic, raw, choice	0
Liver	0
Pastrami, turkey	3
Pâté, liver, canned	1
Pheasant, meat and skin, raw	0
Polish sausage, pork	1
Pork chops	0
Pork loin	0
Pork sausage, fresh, raw	0
Rabbit, wild, raw	0
Salami, dry or hard, pork	1
Salami, Genoa, Oscar Mayer	1
Sausage, Italian, pork, raw	0
Squab, meat and skin, raw	0
Steak	0
Turkey, all classes, meat, skin, giblets, and neck, raw	0
Turkey bacon, Louis Rich	2
Turkey, ground, fat-free, raw	0
Turkey sausage, reduced-fat, cooked	8
Veal, lean and fat, raw	0

FOOD ITEM	TOTAL SUGAR EQUIVALENCY
NUTS AND SEEDS	
Almonds	8
Cashews, raw	22
Coconut meat, raw	6
Coconut milk, raw	3
Macadamia nuts, raw	5
Peanuts, see Vegetables and Legumes	
Pecans	4
Pistachio nuts, raw	15
Sunflower seed kernels	9
Walnuts, English	6
SEAFOOD	
Bass, freshwater, raw	0
Caviar, black and red	3
Clam, raw	3
Cod, Atlantic, raw	0
Crab, Alaska king, raw	0
Eel, raw	0
Grouper, raw	0
Haddock, raw	0
Halibut, raw	0
Herring, Atlantic, raw	0
Lobster, northern, raw	0
Mackerel, Atlantic, raw	0
Oyster, Eastern, wild, raw	2
Perch, ocean, Atlantic, raw	0
Salmon, chinook, raw	0
Scallop, raw	2
Shrimp, raw	1
Sturgeon, raw	0
Swordfish, raw	0
Trout, raw	0
Tuna, fresh, bluefin, raw	0
Tuna, white, canned in oil, drained	0
Tuna, white, canned in water, drained	0

FOOD ITEM	TOTAL SUGAR EQUIVALENCY
VEGETABLES AND LEGUMES	
Artichokes, raw	4
Asparagus, raw	2
Beans, baked, home prepared	12
Beans, lima, baby, raw	12
Beans, lima, raw	35
Beans, kidney, raw	27
Beans, kidney, sprouted, raw	3
Beans, navy, raw	28
Beans, navy, sprouted, raw	10
Beans, pinto, frozen	20
Beans, snap, green, raw	4
Beets, raw	7
Black-eyed peas, raw	11
Broccoli, raw	3
Brussels sprouts, raw	4
Cabbage, raw	3
Carrots, raw	6
Cassava, raw	28
Cauliflower, green, raw	3
Cauliflower, raw	3
Celery, raw	2
Corn, sweet, yellow, raw	14
Cucumber, with peel, raw	3
Eggplant, raw	2
Endive, raw	0
Garlic, raw	23
Ginger root, raw	12
Kale, boiled and drained	3
Lentils, sprouted, raw	17
Lettuce, green leaf, raw	1
Lettuce, iceberg, raw	2
Mushrooms, chanterelle, raw	3
Mushrooms, white, raw	2
Okra, raw	3

FOOD ITEM	TOTAL SUGAR EQUIVALENCY
Onion rings, breaded, frozen	28
Onions, raw	7
Parsley, fresh	2
Peanut butter, smooth or chunky	12
Peanut butter, smooth, reduced-fat	25
Peanuts, all types, raw	7
Peanuts, Spanish, raw	5
Peas, edible-pod, raw	5
Peppers, hot chile, red, raw	7
Peppers, sweet, red, raw	4
Pickle relish	23
Potatoes, baked, flesh and skin	29
Potatoes, frozen shoestring French fries	18
Potatoes, hash brown, home-prepared	24
Potatoes, mashed, from flakes (no milk or butter)	8
Potatoes, red, flesh and skin, raw	11
Potatoes, russet, flesh and skin, raw	13
Potatoes, white, flesh and skin, raw	10
Radishes, raw	2
Sauerkraut, canned, w/liquid	2
Soybeans, green, raw	5
Spinach, raw	1
Squash, summer, raw	4
Sweet potato, baked in skin	15
Sweet potato, raw	14
Tomato products, canned sauce	4
Tomato products, canned sauce, w/mushrooms	7
Tomatoes, red, ripe	3
Turnips, raw	4
Yam, Hawaii, Mountain, raw	12
Yam, raw	18

RESOURCES

Below is a list of additional resources that might be useful when reducing your intake of sugars and other carbohydrates.

Food Addiction: Inspirational Accounts, Research, and Support

Dealing with Food Addiction
> dealingwithfoodaddiction.blogspot.com
> A blog documenting one woman's struggles with obesity and overeating.

Diary of a Former Food Addict
> diaryofaformerfoodaddict.blogspot.com
> A look at the trials, successes, and everyday life of a food addict.

Dr. Avena's Research Website
> drnicoleavena.com
> Dr. Avena's website contains articles and stories about the food addiction and appetite research that is being conducted in her laboratory.

Food Addiction Institute (FAI)
> foodaddictioninstitute.org
> Lists a number of food-addiction and compulsive-eating support groups and meetings, and discusses research regarding food addiction. This website also offers a subscription to their online newsletter and a wide range of suggested books.

Food Addiction Research Education (FARE)
> foodaddictionresearch.org
> Provides Q&A about food addiction, including questions about the withdrawal process, cravings, and how to overcome food addiction. This website also features relevant research findings and news information regarding food addiction.

Food Addicts (FA)

foodaddicts.org

This website can help you find FA meetings, features stories of recovery, includes a section on food addiction in the news, and can be used to subscribe to the FA magazine, *Connection*.

Food Addicts Anonymous (FAA)

foodaddictsanonymous.org

This website can help you find FAA meetings—in person, online, or via telephone—and features testimonials from recovering food addicts.

Food Junkie (Dr. Avena's blog):

psychologytoday.com/blog/food-junkie

Provides a simple-to-understand account of the science behind food addiction.

Overeaters Anonymous (OA)

overeatersanonymous.org

This website can help you find OA meetings and includes many other helpful features, including inspirational podcasts.

Promise of Recovery

promiseofrecovery.com/tag/food-addict-blog

A member of Overeating Anonymous shares her spiritual approach to dealing with her struggles with overeating.

Healthy Lifestyle Tips

A Weigh Out

aweighout.com

Includes information about compulsive and emotional eating, such as podcasts for compulsive and binge eaters, and offers phone seminars.

Choose My Plate

choosemyplate.gov

A project started by the US government's Center for Nutrition Policy and Promotion to promote better nutrition and well-being among Americans. This website includes tips on how to eat healthy on a budget, a BMI calculator, nutrition information for thousands of food items, and trackers for food intake, physical activity, and goals.

First Ourselves
firstourselves.org
Includes support and guidance for bingeing, food cravings, sugar addiction, body image, weight loss, and more. Also includes a discussion forum.

Normal Eating
normaleating.com
Features an online forum that offers information and support for emotional eaters and features a test to see why you may eat.

Spark People
sparkpeople.com
Offers nutrition, health, and fitness tools, support, and resources, including food and fitness trackers.

Sugar-Free and Low-Carb Living: Inspiration and Recipes

Carbohydrate Counter
carbohydrate-counter.org
Find out the carbohydrate content of many common foods.

Diabetic-Friendly Recipes
cooksrecipes.com/category/diabetic.html
Tons of free recipes!

Diet Grail
dietgrail.com/sugars
Find out the sugar content and glycemic index of many common foods.

George Stella's Low-Carb Community
stellastyle.com
Includes a family's weight-loss story, how-to guide for low-carb diets, and low-carb recipes.

Going Sugar Free: Delicious Eats without Artificial Sweets
goingsugarfree.com

Includes recipes and helpful hints on sugar substitutions, lists products on the market with little to no sugar, and explains the various names of sugar that you may come across when reading a nutrition label.

Livin' La Vida Low-Carb
livinlavidalowcarb.com/blog

Jimmy Moore's personal account of his discovery of a low-carb lifestyle.

My Years Without Sugar
myyearwithout.blogspot.com

Documents a personal quest to live on a sugar-free diet.

Sarah Wilson
sarahwilson.com.au

Offers recipes and ebooks, like the *I Quit Sugar Cookbook*.

Simply Sugar and Gluten Free
simplysugarandglutenfree.com

In addition to recipes, this website includes a list of helpful ingredient substitutions.

Spoonful of Sugar Free
spoonfulofsugarfree.com

Includes a new sugar-, dairy-, and gluten-free recipe each day.

Sugar Stacks
sugarstacks.com

A helpful site for visualizing how much sugar is contained in various foods.

USDA National Nutrient Database
ndb.nal.usda.gov/ndb/search/list

Searchable database compiled by the USDA regarding the nutrient, calorie, carbohydrate, and sugar content in foods.

ENDNOTES

Introduction

1. Flegal K, Carroll M, Ogden C, Curtin L (2010). Prevalence and trends in obesity among US adults, 1999–2008. *JAMA* 303(3): 235–41.
2. Finkelstein EA, Khavjou OA, Thompson H, Trogdon JG, Pan L, Sherry B, et al. (2012). Obesity and severe obesity forecasts through 2030. *Am J Prev Med* 42(6): 563–70.
3. Taubes, G (2011, April 17). Is sugar toxic? *New York Times Magazine*: MM47.
4. Taubes G (2011). *Why we get fat: And what to do about it.* New York: Anchor Books.
5. Shai I, Schwarzfuchs D, Henkin Y, Shahar DR, Witkow S, Greenberg I, et al. (2008). Weight loss with a low-carbohydrate, Mediterranean, or low-fat diet. *N Engl J Med* 359(3): 229–41.
6. Astrup A, Meinert Larsen T, Harper A (2004). Atkins and other low-carbohydrate diets: Hoax or an effective tool for weight loss? *Lancet* 364(9437): 897–9.

Step 1: Why Your Past Diet Attempts Have Failed

1. Sikorski C, Riedel C, Luppa M, Schulze B, Werner P, König HH, et al. (2012). Perception of overweight and obesity from different angles: A qualitative study. *Scand J Public Health* 40(3): 271–7.
2. Cecil J, Dalton M, Finlayson G, Blundell J, Hetherington M, Palmer C (2012). Obesity and eating behavior in children and adolescents: Contribution of common gene polymorphisms. *Int Rev Psychiatry* 24(3): 200–10.
3. Neumark-Sztainer D, Wall M, Story M, Standish AR (2012). Dieting and unhealthy weight control behaviors during adolescence: Associations with 10-year changes in body mass index. *J Adolesc Health* 50(1): 80–6.

4. Perri MG, Nezu AM, Patti ET, McCann KL (1989). Effect of length of treatment on weight loss. *J Consult Clin Psychol* 57(3): 450–2.

5. Drewnowski A, Specter SE (2004). Poverty and obesity: The role of energy density and energy costs. *Am J Clin Nutr* 79(1): 6–16.

6. Raynor HA, Kilanowski CK, Esterlis I, Epstein LH (2002). A cost-analysis of adopting a healthful diet in a family-based obesity treatment program. *J Am Diet Assoc* 102(5): 645–56.

7. Sonneville KR, La Pelle N, Taveras EM, Gillman MW, Prosser LA (2009). Economic and other barriers to adopting recommendations to prevent childhood obesity: Results of a focus group study with parents. *BMC Pediatrics* 9: 81.

8. Christie C (2010). Maintaining a heart-healthy diet most of the time. *Journal of Cardiovascular Nursing* 25(3): 233.

9. Centers for Disease Control and Prevention (2011). How much physical activity do adults need? Accessed 30 Mar 2013, http://www.cdc.gov/physicalactivity/everyone/guidelines/adults.html.

10. Centers for Disease Control and Prevention (2011). Overcoming barriers to physical activity. Accessed 30 Mar 2013, http://www.cdc.gov/physicalactivity/everyone/getactive/barriers.html.

11. "Atkins survey finds Americans are confused about carbohydrates" (2012). Retrieved from http://www.atkins.com/Library/Press-Releases/2012/Atkins-Survey-Finds-Americans-Are-Confused-About-C.aspx. Accessed May 5, 2013.

12. Shai I, Schwarzfuchs D, Henkin Y, Shahar DR, Witkow S, Greenberg I, et al. (2008). Weight loss with a low-carbohydrate, Mediterranean, or low-fat diet. *N Engl J Med* 359(3): 229–41.

13. Brehm BJ, Seeley RJ, Daniels SR, D'Alessio DA (2003). A randomized trial comparing a very low carbohydrate diet and a calorie-restricted low fat diet on body weight and cardiovascular risk factors in healthy women. *J Clin Endocrinol Metab* 88(4): 1617–23.

14. "Atkins survey finds Americans are confused about carbohydrates" (2012). Retrieved from http://www.atkins.com/Library/Press-Releases/2012/Atkins-Survey-Finds-Americans-Are-Confused-About-C.aspx. Accessed May 5, 2013.

15. Ibid.

Step 2: Weigh In on Your Sugar Intake

1. USDA Center for Nutrition Policy and Promotion (2011). A brief history of USDA food guides. Retrieved from www.choosemyplate.gov/food-groups/downloads/MyPlate/ABriefHistoryOfUSDAFoodGuides.pdf. Accessed May 5, 2013.
2. Roberts S (2000). High-glycemic index foods, hunger, and obesity: Is there a connection? *Nutr Rev* 58(6): 163–9.
3. Beulens JW, de Bruijne LM, Stolk RP, Peeters PH, Bots ML, Grobbee DE, et al. (2007). High dietary glycemic load and glycemic index increase risk of cardiovascular disease among middle-aged women. *J Am Coll Cardio* 50(1): 14–21.
4. Willett W, Manson J, Liu S (2002). Glycemic index, glycemic load, and risk of type 2 diabetes. *Am J Clin Nutr* 76(1): 274S–80S.
5. Rothman RL, Housam R, Weiss H, Davis D, Gregory R, Gebretsadik T, et al. (2006). Patient understanding of food labels: The role of literacy and numeracy. *Am J of Prev Med* 31(5): 391–8.
6. Johnson RK, Yon BA (2010). Weighing in on added sugars and health. *J Am Diet Assoc* 110(9): 1296–9.
7. Young LR, Nestle M (2002). The contribution of expanding portion sizes to the US obesity epidemic. *Am J Public Health* 92: 246–9.
8. Nielsen SJ, Popkin BM (2003). Patterns and trends in food portion sizes, 1977–1998. *JAMA* 289: 450–3.
9. Rolls BJ, Morris EL, Roe LS (2002). Portion size and food affects energy intake in normal-weight and overweight men and women. *Am J Clin Nutr* 7(6): 1207–13.
10. American Institute for Cancer Research (2003). *Awareness and action: AICR surveys on portion size, nutrition, and cancer risk*. Washington, DC.
11. Wansink B, van Ittersum K (2007). Portion size me: Down-sizing our consumption norms. *J Am Diet Assoc* 10(7): 1103–6.
12. Lin B-H, Guthrie J, Frazão E (1999). Chapter 12: Nutrient contribution of food away from home. AIB-750. United States Department of Agriculture. Retrieved from http://ers.usda.gov/media/91062/aib750l_1_.pdf. Accessed May 5, 2013.

Step 3: The New Science of Sugar Addiction

1. Karim R, Chaudhri P (2012). Behavioral addictions: An overview. *J Psychoactive Drugs* 44(1): 5–17.

2. Alcoholics Anonymous of Akron, Ohio (n.d.). *Manual for alcoholics anonymous* (5th ed.). Akron, OH, 21.

3. Kampov-Polevoy AB, Garbutt JC, Janowsky DS (1999). Association between preference for sweets and excessive alcohol intake: A review of animal and human studies. *Alcohol* 34(3): 386–95.

4. Dotson CD, Spector AC (2004). The relative affective potency of glycine, L-serine and sucrose as assessed by a brief-access taste test in inbred strains of mice. *Chem Senses* 29(6): 489–98.

5. Ren X, Ferreira JG, Zhou L, Shammah-Lagnado SJ, Yeckel CW, de Araujo IE (2010). Nutrient selection in the absence of taste receptor signaling. *J Neurosci* 30(23): 8012–23.

6. Ibid.

7. Ibid.

8. Aston-Jones G, Smith RJ, Sartor GC, Moorman DE, Massi L, Tahsili-Fahadan P, Richardson KA (2010). Lateral hypothalamic orexin/hypocretin neurons: A role in reward-seeking and addiction. *Brain Res* 1314: 74–90.

9. Fulton S, Pissios P, Manchon RP, Stiles L, Frank L, Pothos EN, et al. (2006). Leptin regulation of the mesoaccumbens dopamine pathway. *Neuron* 51(6): 811–22.

10. Mebel DM, Wong JC, Dong YJ, Borgland SL (2012). Insulin in the ventral tegmental area reduces hedonic feeding and suppresses dopamine concentration via increased reuptake. *Eur J Neurosci* 36(3): 2336–46.

11. Avena NM, Rada P, Hoebel BG (2008). Evidence for sugar addiction: Behavioral and neurochemical effects of intermittent, excessive sugar intake. *Neurosci Biobehav Rev* 32(1): 20–39.

12. Kampov-Polevoy AB, Garbutt JC, Janowsky DS (1999). Association between preference for sweets and excessive alcohol intake: A review of animal and human studies. *Alcohol* 34(3): 386–95.

13. Avena NM, Rada P, Hoebel BG (2008). Evidence for sugar addiction: Behavioral and neurochemical effects of intermittent, excessive sugar intake. *Neurosci Biobehav Rev* 32(1): 20–39.

14. Oswald KD, Murdaugh DL, King VL, Boggiano MM (2011). Motivation for palatable food despite consequences in an animal model of binge eating. *Int J Eat Disord* 44(3): 203–11.

15. Gearhardt AN, Corbin WR, Brownell KD (2009). Preliminary validation of the Yale Food Addiction Scale. *Appetite* 52(2): 430–6.

16. Ifland JR, Preuss HG, Marcus MT, Rourke KM, Taylor WC, Burau K, et al. (2009). Refined food addiction: A classic substance use disorder. *Med Hypotheses* 72(5): 518–26.

17. Gearhardt AN, Corbin WR, Brownell KD (2009). Preliminary validation of the Yale Food Addiction Scale. *Appetite* 52(2): 430–6.

18. Meule A, Heckel D, Kübler A (2012). Factor structure and item analysis of the Yale Food Addiction Scale in obese candidates for bariatric surgery. *Eur Eat Disord Rev* 20(5): 419–22.

19. Bartholome LT, Raymond NC, Lee SS, Peterson CB, Warren CS (2006). Detailed analysis of binges in obese women with binge eating disorder: Comparisons using multiple methods of data collection. *Int J Eat Disord* 39(8): 685–93.

20. Gearhardt AN, Yokum S, Orr PT, Stice E, Corbin WR, Brownell KD (2011). Neural correlates of food addiction. *Arch Gen Psychiatry* 68(8): 808–16.

21. Lim HK, Pae CU, Joo RH, Yoo SS, Choi BG, Kim DJ, et al. (2005). fMRI investigation on cue-induced smoking craving. *J Psychiatr Res* 39(3): 333–5.

22. Engelmann JM, Versace F, Robinson JD, Minnix JA, Lam CY, Cui Y, et al. (2012). Neural substrates of smoking cue reactivity: A meta-analysis of fMRI studies. *Neuroimage* 60(1): 252–62.

23. Wang GJ, Volkow ND, Logan J, Pappas NR, Wong CT, Zhu W, et al. (2001). Brain dopamine and obesity. *Lancet* 357(9253): 354–7.

24. Verbeken S, Braet C, Lemmertyn J, Goossens L, Moens E (2012). How is reward sensitivity related to bodyweight in children? *Appetite* 58(2): 478–83.

25. Ibid.

26. Ibid.

27. Davis C, Fox J (2008). Sensitivity to reward and body mass index (BMI): Evidence for a non-linear relationship. *Appetite* 50(1): 43–49.

28. Gearhardt AN, Yokum S, Orr PT, Stice E, Corbin WR, Brownell KD (2011). Neural correlates of food addiction. *Arch Gen Psychiatry* 68(8): 808–16.

29. Berridge KC, Robinson TE, Aldridge JW (2009). Dissecting components of reward: "Liking,", "wanting," and learning. *Curr Opin Pharmacol* 9(1): 65–73.

30. Lennerz BS, Alsop DC, Holsen LM, Stern E, Rojas R, Ebbeling CB, et al. (2013). Effects of dietary glycemic index on brain regions related to reward and craving in men. *Am J Clin Nutr*: Epub ahead of print.

Step 4: The Sugar Freedom Plan for Breaking Your Addiction

1. Ebbeling CB, Swain JF, Feldman HA, Wong WW, Hachey DL, Garcia-Lago E, Ludwig DS (2012). Effects of dietary composition on energy expenditure during weight-loss maintenance. *JAMA* 307(24): 2627–34.

2. O'Keefe JH, Gheewala NM, O'Keefe JO (2008). Dietary strategies for improving post-prandial glucose, lipids, inflammation, and cardiovascular health. *J Am Coll Cardiol* 51(3): 249–55.

3. Popkin BM (2012). Sugary beverages represent a threat to global health. *Trends Endocrinol Metab* 23(12): 591–3.

4. Malik VS, Popkin BM, Bray GA, Després JP, Willett WC, Hu FB (2010). Sugar-sweetened beverages and risk of metabolic syndrome and type 2 diabetes. *Diabetes Care* 33(11): 2477–83.

5. Popkin BM (2012). The changing face of global diet and nutrition. In *Food and addiction: A comprehensive handbook.* Oxford University Press, 69–80. Edited by KD Brownell and MS Gold.

6. Mattes RD (1996). Dietary compensation by humans for supplemental energy provided as ethanol or carbohydrate in fluids. *Physiol Behav* 59(1): 179–87.

7. Di Meglio DP, Mattes RD (2000). Liquid versus solid carbohydrate: Effects on food intake and body weight. *Int J Obes Relat Metab Disord* 24(6): 794–800.

8. Chen L, Appel LJ, Loria C, Lin PH, Champagne CM, Elmer PJ, et al. (2009). Reduction in consumption of sugar-sweetened beverages is associated with weight loss: The PREMIER trial. *Am J Clin Nutr* 89(5): 1299–1306.

9. Centers for Disease Control and Prevention (2011). NCHS data brief: Consumption of sugar drinks in the United States, 2005–2008. Retrieved from www.cdc.gov/nchs/data/databriefs/db71.htm. Accessed May 5, 2013.

10. Wang YC, Coxson P, Shen YM, Goldman L, Bibbins-Domingo K (2012). A penny-per-ounce tax on sugar-sweetened beverages would cut health and cost burdens of diabetes. *Health Aff* 31(1): 199–207.

11. Ebbling CA, Willett, WC, Ludwig DS (2012). The special case of sugar-sweetened beverages. In *Food and addiction: A comprehensive handbook.* Oxford University Press, 147–53. Edited by KD Brownell and MS Gold.

12. Vivar C, Potter MC, van Praag H (2012). All about running: Synaptic plasticity, growth factors, and adult hippocampal neurogenesis. *Curr Top Behav Neurosci* (Epub ahead of print).

13. Salmon P (2001). Effects of physical exercise on anxiety, depression, and sensitivity to stress: A unifying theory. *Clin Psychol Rev* 21(1): 33–61.

14. Howlett TA, Tomlin S, Ngahfoong L, Rees LH, Bullen BA, Skrinar GS, McArthur JW (1984). Release of beta endorphin and met-enkephalin during exercise in normal women: Response to training. *Br Med J (Clin Res Ed)* 288(6435): 1950–2.

15. Jamurtas AZ, Tofas T, Fatouros I, Nikolaidis MG, Paschalis V, Yfanti C, et al. (2011). The effects of low and high glycemic index foods on exercise performance and beta-endorphin responses. *J Int Soc Sports Nutr* 8: 15.

16. Ivezaj V, Saules KK, Wiedemann AA (2012). "I didn't see this coming": Why are postbariatric patients in substance abuse treatment? Patients' perceptions of etiology and future recommendations. *Obes Surg* 22(8): 1308–14.

17. King WC, Chen JY, Mitchell JE, Kalarchian MA, Steffen KJ, Engel SG, et al. (2012). Prevalence of alcohol use disorders before and after bariatric surgery. *JAMA* 307(23): 2516–25.

18. Lindqvist A, de la Cour CD, Stegmark A, Håkanson R, Erlanson-Albertsson C (2005). Overeating of palatable food is associated with blunted leptin and ghrelin responses. *Regul Pept* 130(3): 123–32.

19. Halton TL, Hu FB (2004). The effects of high protein diets on thermogenesis, satiety, and weight loss: A critical review. *J Am Coll Nutr* 23(5): 373–85.

Step 5: What to Eat and What *Not* to Eat

1. Di Meglio DP, Mattes RD (2000). Liquid versus solid carbohydrate: Effects on food intake and body weight. *Int J Obes Relat Metab Disord* 24(6): 794–800.

2. Sclafani A, Ackroff K (1994). Glucose- and fructose-conditioned flavor preferences in rats: Taste versus postingestive conditioning. *Physiol Behav* 56(2): 399–405.

3. Soffritti M, Belpoggi F, Tibaldi E, Esposti DD, Lauriola M (2007). Life-span exposure to low doses of aspartame beginning during prenatal life increases cancer effects in rats. *Environ Health Perspect* 115(9): 1293–7.

4. Bryan GT, Erturk E, Yoshida O (1970). Production of urinary bladder carcinomas in mice by sodium saccharin. *Science* 168(3936): 1238–40.

5. Patel RM, Sarma R, Grimsley E (2006). Popular sweetener sucralose as a migraine trigger. *Headache* 46(8): 1303–4.

6. American Cancer Society (2011). Aspartame. Retrieved from http://www.cancer.org/Cancer/CancerCauses/OtherCarcinogens/AtHome/aspartame. Accessed May 5, 2013.

7. St-Onge MP, Heymsfield SB (2003). Usefulness of artificial sweeteners for body weight control. *Nutr Rev* 61(6 Pt 1): 219–21.

8. Gardner C, Wylie-Rosett J, Gidding SS, Steffen LM, Johnson RK, Reader D, et al.; American Heart Association Nutrition Committee of the Council on Nutrition, Physical Activity and Metabolism, Council on Arteriosclerosis, Thrombosis and Vascular Biology, Council on Cardiovascular Disease in the Young; American Diabetes Association (2012). Nonnutritive sweeteners: Current use and health perspectives: A scientific statement from the American Heart Association and the American Diabetes Association. *Diabetes Care* 35(8): 1798–1808.

9. Gibson SA, Gunn P (2011). What's for breakfast? Nutritional implications of breakfast habits: Insights from the NDNS dietary records. *Nutrition Bulletin* 36(1): 78–86.

10. Cooper SB, Bandelow S, Nevill ME (2011). Breakfast consumption and cognitive function in adolescent schoolchildren. *Physiol Behav* 103(5): 431–9.

11. Affenito SG (2007). Breakfast: A missed opportunity. *J Am Diet Assoc* 107(4): 565–9.

12. Huang CJ, Hu HT, Fan YC, Liao YM, Tsai PS (2010). Associations of breakfast skipping with obesity and health-related quality of life: Evidence from a national survey in Taiwan. *Int J Obes* 34(4): 720–5.

13. Kayman S, Bruvold W, Stern JS (1990). Maintenance and relapse after weight loss in women: Behavioral aspects. *Am J Clin Nutr* 52(5): 800–7.

14. Duffey KJ, Popkin BM (2011). Energy density, portion size, and eating occasions: Contributions to increased energy intake in the United States, 1977–2006. *PLoS Med* 8(6): e1001050.

15. Ibid.

16. Furchner-Evanson A, Petrisko Y, Howarth L, Nemoseck T, Kern M (2010). Type of snack influences satiety responses in adult women. *Appetite* 54(3): 564–9.

Step 6: Managing Your Withdrawal

1. Avena NM, Rada P, Hoebel BG (2008). Evidence for sugar addiction: Behavioral and neurochemical effects of intermittent, excessive sugar intake. *Neurosci Biobehav Rev* 32(1): 20–39.

2. Ziauddeen H, Farooqi IS, Fletcher PC (2012). Obesity and the brain: How convincing is the addiction model? *Nat Rev Neurosci* 13(4): 279–86.
3. Crews FT, Boettiger CA (2009). Impulsivity, frontal lobes, and risk for addiction. *Pharmacol Biochem Behav* 93(3): 237–47.
4. West R, Gossop M (1994). Overview: A comparison of withdrawal symptoms from different drug classes. *Addiction* 89(11): 1483–9.
5. Ifland JR, Preuss HG, Marcus MT, Rourke KM, Taylor WC, Burau K, et al. (2009). Refined food addiction: A classic substance use disorder. *Med Hypotheses* 72(5): 518–26.
6. Avena NM, Rada P, Hoebel BG (2008). Evidence for sugar addiction: Behavioral and neurochemical effects of intermittent, excessive sugar intake. *Neurosci Biobehav Rev* 32(1): 20–39.
7. Hall DM, Most MM (2005). Dietary adherence in well-controlled feeding studies. *J Am Diet Assoc* 105(8): 1285–8.
8. Mayo Clinic (2011). Quitting smoking: 10 ways to resist tobacco cravings. Retrieved from http://www.mayoclinic.com/health/nicotine-craving/SK00057. Accessed May 5, 2013.
9. Best DW, Lubman DI (2012). The recovery paradigm: A model of hope and change for alcohol and drug addiction. *Australian Family Physician* 41(8): 593–97.
10. Sobell LC, Ellingstad TP, Sobell MB (2000). Natural recovery from alcohol and drug problems: Methodological review of the research with suggestions for future directions. *Addiction* 95(5): 749–64.
11. Davis W (2011). *Wheat belly.* New York: Rodale.
12. Griswell JB, Jennings B (2009). *The adversity paradox: An unconventional guide to achieving uncommon business success.* New York: St. Martin's Press.

Step 7: Managing Your Cravings

1. Weingarten HP, Elston D (1991). Food cravings in a college population. *Appetite* 173(3): 167–75.
2. Lappalainen R, Sjoden PO, Hursti T, Vesa V (1990). Hunger/craving responses and reactivity to food stimuli during fasting and dieting. *Int J Obes* 14(8): 679–88.
3. Harvey J, Wing RR, Mullen M (1993). Effects on food cravings of a very low calorie diet or a balanced, low calorie diet. *Appetite* 21(2): 105–15.
4. Massey A, Hill AJ (2012). Dieting and food craving: A descriptive, quasi-prospective study. *Appetite* 58(3): 781–5.

5. Gilhooly CH, Das SK, Golden JK, McCrory MA, Dallal GE, Saltzman E, et al. (2007). Food cravings and energy regulation: The characteristics of craved foods and their relationship with eating behaviors and weight change during 6 months of dietary energy restriction. *Int J Obes* 31(12): 1849–58.

6. Martin CK, Rosenbaum D, Han H, Geiselman PJ, Wyatt HR, Hill JO, et al. (2011). Change in food cravings, food preferences, and appetite during a low-carbohydrate and low-fat diet. *Obesity* 19(10): 1963–70.

7. United States Department of Agriculture (2003). *Agriculture fact book, 2001–2002*. Chapter 2: Profiling food consumption in America. Retrieved from http://usinfo.org/enus/economy/industry/docs/2002factbook.pdf. Accessed May 5, 2013.

8. Elkort M (1991). *The secret life of food: A feast of food and drink history, folklore, and fact*. Los Angeles: J. P. Tarcher.

9. Hall DM, Most MM (2005). Dietary adherence in well-controlled feeding studies. *J Am Diet Assoc* 105(8): 1285–8.

10. United States Department of Agriculture (2003). *Agriculture fact book, 2001–2002*. Chapter 2: Profiling food consumption in America. Retrieved from http://usinfo.org/enus/economy/industry/docs/2002factbook.pdf. Accessed May 5, 2013.

11. Ibid.

12. Oliver G, Wardle J, Gibson EL (2000). Stress and food choice: A laboratory study. *Psychosom Med* 62(6): 853–65.

13. Torres SJ, Nowson CA (2007). Relationship between stress, eating behavior, and obesity. *Nutrition* 23(11–12): 887–94.

14. Adam TC, Epel ES (2007). Stress, eating, and the reward system. *Physiol Behav* 91(4): 449–58.

15. Zellner DA, Loaiza S, Gonzalez Z, Pita J, Morales J, Pecora D, et al. (2006). Food selection changes under stress. *Physiol Behav* 87(4): 789–93.

16. Lim SS, Norman RJ, Clifton PM, Noakes M (2009). Hyperandrogenemia, psychological distress, and food cravings in young women. *Physiol Behav* 98(3): 276–80.

17. Ibid.

18. Kandiah J, Yake M, Jones J, Meyer M (2006). Stress influences appetite and comfort food preferences in college women. *Nutrition Res* 26(3): 118–23.

19. Pelchat ML, Johnson A, Chan R, Valdez J, Ragland JD (2004). Images of desire: Food-craving activation during fMRI. *Neuroimage* 23(4): 1486–93.

20. Arredondo E, Castaneda D, Elder JP, Slymen D, Dozier D (2009). Brand name logo recognition of fast food and healthy food among children. *J Community Health* 34(1): 73–78.
21. Rudd Center for Food Policy and Obesity (2010). Evaluating fast food nutrition and marketing to youth. Retrieved from http://www. fastfoodmarketing.org/media/FastFoodFACTS_Report.pdf. Accessed May 5, 2013.
22. Phillips PE, Stuber GD, Heien ML, Wightman RM, Carelli RM (2003). Subsecond dopamine release promotes cocaine seeking. *Nature* 422(6932): 614–8.
23. Li Q, Wang Y, Zhang Y, Li W, Yang W, Zhu J, et al. (2012). Craving correlates with mesolimbic responses to heroin-related cues in short-term abstinence from heroin: An event-related fMRI study. *Brain Res* 1469: 63–72.
24. Scharmüller W, Übel S, Ebner F, Schienle A (2012). Appetite regulation during food cue exposure: A comparison of normal-weight and obese women. *Neurosci Lett* 518(2): 106–10.
25. Werthmann J, Roefs A, Nederkoorn C, Mogg K, Bradley BP, Jansen A (2011). Can(not) take my eyes off it: Attention bias for food in overweight participants. *Health Psychol* 30(5): 561–9.
26. Mayo Clinic (2011). Quitting smoking: 10 ways to resist tobacco cravings. Retrieved from http://www.mayoclinic.com/health/nicotine-craving/SK00057. Accessed May 5, 2013.

Step 8: Avoiding a Relapse

1. Byrne SM, Cooper Z, Fairburn CG (2004). Psychological predictors of weight regain in obesity. *Behav Res Ther* 42(11): 1341–56.
2. Niemeier HM, Phelan S, Fava JL, Wing RR (2007). Internal disinhibition predicts weight regain following weight loss and weight loss maintenance. *Obesity* 15(10): 2485–94.
3. Kayman S, Bruvold W, Stern JS (1990). Maintenance and relapse after weight loss in women: Behavioral aspects. *Am J Clin Nutr* 52(5): 800–7.
4. Ibid.
5. Hendershot CS, Witkiewitz K, George WH, Marlatt GA (2011). Relapse prevention for addictive behaviors. *Subst Abuse Treat Prev Policy* 6: 17.
6. Kayman S, Bruvold W, Stern JS (1990). Maintenance and relapse after weight loss in women: Behavioral aspects. *Am J Clin Nutr* 52(5): 800–7.
7. Ibid.
8. Ibid.

9. Byrne SM, Cooper Z, Fairburn CG (2004). Psychological predictors of weight regain in obesity. *Behav Res Ther* 42(11): 1341–56.

Conclusion: How to Maintain Your New, Addiction-Free Way of Eating

1. Cordain L (2011). *The paleo diet.* Hoboken, NJ: John Wiley & Sons.
2. Bohay M, Blakely DP, Tamplin AK, Radvansky GA (2011). Note taking, review, memory, and comprehension. *Am J Psychol* 124(1): 63–73.
3. Stroebe W, Mensink W, Aarts H, Schut H, Kruglanski AW (2008). Why dieters fail: Testing the goal conflict model of eating. *J Exp Soc Psychol* 44: 26–36.
4. Shah JY, Friedman R, Kruglanski AW (2002). Forgetting all else: On the antecedents and consequences of goal shielding. *J Pers Soc Psychol* 83(6): 1261–80.
5. Pachucki MA, Jacques PF, Christakis NA (2011). Social network concordance in food choice among spouses, friends, and siblings. *Am J Public Health* 101(11): 2170–7.
6. Morland K, Wing S, Diez Roux A (2002). The contextual effect of the local food environment on residents' diets: The Atherosclerosis Risk in Communities Study. *Am J Public Health* 92(11): 1761–7.
7. French SA, Story M, Fulkerson JA, Gerlach AF (2003). Food environment in secondary schools: Á la carte, vending machines, and food policies and practices. *Am J Public Health* 93(7): 1161–7.
8. De Castro JM (1994). Family and friends produce greater social facilitation of food intake than other companions. *Physiol Behav* 56(3): 445–5.
9. Stroebele N, De Castro JM (2004). Effect of ambience on food intake and food choice. *Nutrition* 20(9): 821–38.
10. Kearney MH (1998). Truthful self-nurturing: A grounded formal theory of women's addiction recovery. *Qual Health Res* 8(4): 495–512.
11. Adam TC, Epel ES (2007). Stress, eating, and the reward system. *Physiol Behav* 91(4): 449–58.
12. Macht M (1999). Characteristics of eating in anger, fear, sadness, and joy. *Appetite* 33(1): 129–39.
13. Taheri S, Lin L, Austin D, Young T, Mignot E (2004). Short sleep duration is associated with reduced leptin, elevated ghrelin, and increased body mass index. *PLoS Med* 1(3): e62.

14. Benedict C, Brooks SJ, O'Daly OG, Almèn MS, Morell A, Åberg K, et al. (2012). Acute sleep deprivation enhances the brain's response to hedonic food stimuli: An fMRI study. *J Clin Endocrinol Metab* 97(3): E443–7.

15. St-Onge MP, McReynolds A, Trivedi ZB, Roberts AL, Sy M, Hirsch J (2012). Sleep restriction leads to increased activation of brain regions sensitive to food stimuli. *Am J Clin Nutr* 95(4): 818–24.

16. Taheri S, Lin L, Austin D, Young T, Mignot E (2004). Short sleep duration is associated with reduced leptin, elevated ghrelin, and increased body mass index. *PLoS Med* 1(3): e62.

17. Hammond M (2007). Mindful eating. Tuning in to your food. *Diabetes Self Manag* 24(2): 36, 38, 40.

18. Chozen Bays J (2009). *Mindful eating: A guide to rediscovering a healthy and joyful relationship with food.* Boston: Shambhala Publications.

19. Albers S (2012). *Eating mindfully: How to end mindless eating and enjoy a balanced relationship with food* (2nd ed.). Oakland, CA: New Harbinger Publications.

20. Wing RR, Phelan S (2005). Long-term weight loss maintenance. *Am J Clin Nutr* 82(1): 222S–5S.

INDEX

A

Acetylcholine, 64
Addiction
    boredom and, 110–11
    brain systems involved in,
        62–65
    causes of, 11–12, 185–86
    cross-sensitization and, 71–72
    cycle of, 61, 142
    diagnostic criteria for, 59–60
    guilt and, 191–92
    opponent-process theory of,
        144–45
    personal responsibility and, 20
    power of, 141–43
    symptoms of, 60
    tolerance and, 46, 61
    willpower and, 142
    See also Food addiction;
        Relapse; Withdrawal
Addiction transfer, 114
The Adversity Paradox (Griswell
    and Jennings), 151
American Cancer Society, 124
American Diabetes Association,
    91, 124
American Heart Association,
    51, 124
Artificial sweeteners, 122–25
Aspartame, 122, 123, 124
Atkins Diet, 13

B

Beans, 126, 202
Beverages, 99–101, 120–22, 201
Binges, 61, 70–71
Black-and-white thinking, 167–68
Blame, 19–20
Blood sugar levels, 37, 104
BMI (body mass index), 22
Boredom, 110–11
Breads
    low-carbohydrate, 96
    at restaurants, 180
    sugar equivalency of, 95–96, 202
Breakfast, 132–34
Butter, 198

C

Cakes, 95, 202
Calories
    counting, 112
    empty, 33, 38
Candies, 95, 203–5
Carbohydrates
    counting, 30, 91–92
    fast vs. slow, 37
    reducing, 30–31, 38, 91, 103–5
    simple vs. complex, 36–37, 104
Centers for Disease Control and
    Prevention (CDC), 27–28
Cereals, 95, 96, 199

Cheese, 95, 129, 197
Chocolate, 204
Coffee, 120, 121, 201
Cold turkey, going, 88
Condiments, 130
Conditioning, classical, 159–61
Consistency, importance of,
    190–91
Cookies
    sugar equivalency of, 95, 202–3
    sugar-free, 106
Corn, 125, 127, 200
Cortisol, 157
Cravings
    combating, 155–58, 163
    definition of, 152
    dieting and, 153
    duration of, 154
    effects of, on brain activity, 158
    emotions and, 157–58
    food cues and, 159–62
    hunger vs., 152–53
    as obstacle to weight loss,
        154, 155
    variety and, 158
Cross-sensitization, 71–72
Cues, 71, 159–62

D

Dairy products, 197–98
Deprivation, feelings of, 170
Desserts, 138–39
Dichotomous thinking, 167–68
Diets
    Atkins, 13
    costs of, 26
    cravings and, 153
    definition of, 21

fad, 29
failure of, 3, 17–22
governmental guidelines for,
    32–33, 34
hunger and, 25
individualizing, 170
as industry, 2, 3
low-carbohydrate, 30–31, 91
low-fat, 29, 30, 116
Mediterranean-style, 30
Paleo, 176
problems with, 24–31
as quick fixes, 22–24
as temporary process, 21–22
2,000-calorie, 44–45
typical first week of, 19
    See also Sugar Freedom Plan
Dinner, 132, 134–36
Dopamine, 63–64, 68–69,
    72–74, 79
Doughnuts, 203
Dynamic vulnerability theory, 79

E

Eggs, 95, 134, 198
Emotions
    cravings and, 157–58
    managing, 168–69, 186, 187–88
Exercise, 27–29, 112–15

F

Family
    reducing sugars for, 97–98
    resistance by, 98, 148–49
    support of, 148
Fast food
    avoiding, 181

conditioning and, 160–61
sugar equivalency of, 95, 205–6
Fats
reducing, 29, 30, 115–16
sugar equivalency of, 93, 198
FDA (Food and Drug
Administration), 29, 32,
41, 124
Fiber, 50
Fish, 129, 201–2
Food addiction
addiction transfer and, 114
brain activation and, 78–81
causes of, 11–12, 185–86
criteria for, 75–76
drug addiction vs., 65–66
power of, 140–41
quitting cold turkey, 88
quiz for, 77
research on, 8, 9, 11–13, 66–76,
78–81
satiety signals and, 112, 115
sharing information about,
183–84
theories of, 79–80
See also Relapse; Withdrawal
Food cues, 71, 159–62
Food diary, keeping, 54–57
Food environment
effects of, 182–83, 186
prevalence of sugar in, 99, 108,
109, 119
Food plate guidelines, 32–33, 34
Food pushers, resisting, 181–84
Food pyramid, 32–33, 34
Friends
eating with, 181–84
opposition from, 148–49
support of, 148

Fruits
benefits of, 50, 127–28
dried, 95, 122, 128, 129, 137
fiber in, 50
juices, 122
as snacks, 137
sugar equivalency of, 95,
128–29, 199–200

G

Gateway effect, 71
Glucose, 36, 39
Glycemic index, 37–38
Glycogen, 36
Goal conflict model of eating, 182
Goals
revising, 171
setting, 188–90
Grains, 205
Griswell, J. Barry, 151
Guilt, 191–92

H

Hunger
cravings vs., 152–53
dieting and, 25
pre-eating and, 137
satiety signals and, 69, 112, 115
Hyperresponsiveness model, 79

I

Ice cream, 46–47, 205
Ingredients list, 43–44
Insulin, 37, 69

J

Jennings, Bob, 151
Junk foods
alternatives to, 125–30, 156–57
average annual consumption
of, 154
eliminating, 102–3
sugar equivalency of, 202–5

K

Kitchen, restocking, 97–98

L

Labels, reading, 40–45
Leptin, 69
Lunch, 132, 134–36

M

Maintenance
importance of, 87, 107, 175, 190
tips for, 109–10, 177–91
Meals
tips for preparing, 28
typical, on Sugar Freedom Plan,
131–39
Meats, 95, 129, 198–99
Mediterranean-style diet, 30
Milk, 95, 121, 197
Mindfulness, 187
Muffins, 203

N

Neotame, 123
Neurotransmitters, 63
Nutrition labels, reading, 40–45
Nuts, 95, 138, 201

O

Obesity
artificial sweeteners and, 124
causes of, 20
epidemic of, 1, 8, 99
genetics and, 21
health risks of, 1
Oils, 95, 198
Opioids, 64
Opponent-process theory, 144–45
Orexin, 69
Overeating
addiction and, 3–4, 112
emotions and, 168–69, 186,
187–88
sleep and, 187

P

Paleo Diet, 176
Parsnips, 126, 127
Pasta, 95, 96, 205, 206
Pavlov, Ivan, 159
Percent Daily Value (%DV), 41–42
Pies, 203
Pizza, 205
Planning, importance of, 106,
149–50, 163, 179
Portion size, 45–47, 116, 196
Positive phrasing, 189
Potatoes, 95, 126, 127, 200
Poultry, 95, 129, 198–99
Pre-eating, 137
Processed foods, 48, 51
Protein, 129–30

Q

Quiz, 77

R

Recipes, adjusting, 98
Relapse
    definition of, 166
    effects of, 165–66
    factors contributing to, 166,
        167–69
    learning from, 172–73
    preventing, 166–71
Restaurants
    ordering at, 179–81
    sugar equivalency table for,
        206–7
    See also Fast food
Reward deficiency syndrome, 79
Rutabagas, 126

S

Saccharin, 123, 124
Salad dressings, 130, 134, 198
Satiety signals, 69, 112, 115
Sauces, 130, 206
Seafood, 95, 129, 201–2
Seeds, 201
Serotonin, 64
Serving size, 43
Shaping, 23
Shopping, 108–9
Sleep, 187
Snacks
    dangers of, 136–38
    sugar equivalency of, 203–5
    on the Sugar Freedom Plan, 132,
        137, 138
Sodas, 46, 47, 99–101, 120, 201
Soups, 136, 206
Sour cream, 198
Spices, 130

Squash, 125, 127, 201
Stress, 157–58, 168–69, 187–88
Sucralose, 123, 124
Sucrose, 35
Sugar addiction. *See* Food
    addiction
Sugar equivalency
    average, by food group, 95
    calculating, 93, 94, 195
    cutoff points for, 93
    table, 92, 195–207
Sugar Freedom Plan
    benefits of, 116–17, 191–94
    boredom and, 110–11
    core principle of, 87–88
    differences between other diets
        and, 86–87
    gradual nature of, 89
    maintaining, 87, 107, 109–10,
        175, 177–91
    phases of, 85, 89–90, 99–107
    preparatory steps for, 90–98
    starting, 99
    typical meals on, 131–39
    vegetarian options in, 135
Sugar-free foods, 106, 130
Sugars
    added, 44, 51, 95, 156
    in beverages, 99–101, 120–22
    definition of, 35
    eliminating vs. reducing, 108–10
    in fruits, 50
    hidden, 97, 106–7, 130–31
    in popular foods, 47, 49
    sense of taste and, 131
    substitutes for, 122–25
    tracking intake of, 52–53, 54–57
    types of, 39, 40, 95–97
Support, sources of, 148–49
Sweet potatoes, 126, 127, 201

T

Taste, sense of, 131
Taubes, Gary, 4
Tea, 120, 201
Thinking, black-and-white,
    167–68
Tolerance, 46, 61

V

Variety, importance of, 158
Vegetables
    carbohydrate content of, 125–27
    as snacks, 137
    sugar equivalency of, 95,
        200–201
Vegetarian options, 135

W

Water, 120
Weight loss
    artificial sweeteners and, 124
    cravings and, 154, 155
    exercise and, 112–15
    fiber and, 50
    goals for, 171
    hunger and, 25
    inevitability of, 112, 116
    motivations for, 1
    rate of, 23–24

Why We Get Fat (Taubes), 4
Willpower, 142
Withdrawal
    definition of, 144
    exercise and, 113
    length of, 146
    symptoms of, 6–7, 13–14, 62,
        143–46
    tips for managing, 146–51

Y

Yale Food Addiction Scale, 75–76
Yams, 126, 127, 201
Yogurt, 134, 197–98

COOP 10/14